Countertransference and Alive Moments

Help or Hindrance

Help or Hindrance

R.D HINSHELWOOD

Countertransference and Alive Moments
Help or Hindrance

Published by Process Press Ltd.

Text Copyright © 2016 Robert Hinshelwood

All Rights Reserved

ISBN 978-1-899209-17-0

For information on other books written by R.D.Hinshelwood
please go to

www.rdhinshelwood.net

Contents

About the Author..*v*

Acknowledgements ....*vii*

Preface..*ix*

Introduction..*1*

PART 1: IN HISTORICAL TIMES **5**

C H A P T E R 1: *Shame amongst friends*

What could Freud say? 7

C H A P T E R 2: *Distantiation, said Erikson*

What could they all do?.. 15

C H A P T E R 3: *Wanted dead or alive*

What are live moments? 27

PART TWO: PARADIGM SHIFT **37**

C H A P T E R 4: *Ferenczi and British psychoanalysis*
What put British psychoanalysis ahead? 41

C H A P T E R 5: *Unconscious-to-unconscious*
How do they communicate? 51

C H A P T E R 6: *Debate – Klein/Heimann*
What unacknowledged agreement did they reach?.......................... 75

C H A P T E R 7 : *Co-constructed intersubjectivity*
Where did ego-psychology go? 89

C H A P T E R 8 : *Critical debate – Conclusions to Part 2*
How do the trends compare?.. 107

C H A P T E R 9 : *Interlude – The unconscious in Freud*
Can we test the new view?.. 125

PART 3: AT WORK TODAY................................**135**

C H A P T E R 10 : *Enactment*
What's happening?.. 139

C H A P T E R 11 : *The reflective analyst*
What was that? 153

C H A P T E R 12 : *And the reflective patient, also*
What does the patient see? 161

C H A P T E R 13 : *Resisting the death instinct*
What's the difference? 175

PART 4: REACHING BEYOND........................**193**

C H A P T E R 14 : *Morals and ethics*
Who has the authority?.. 197

C H A P T E R 15 : *Research data*
How 'true' is countertransference?........................... 219

C H A P T E R 16 : *Now about the question...* 235

References.. 241

About the Author

Following his medical training at the time of the anti-psychiatry movement, Bob Hinshelwood started working as a psychiatrist in London in 1966. He worked in the NHS for 30 years, as well as having a part-time practice as a psychoanalyst since 1975, when he qualified with the British Psychoanalytical Society. He has contributed to the therapeutic community movement, including taking the role of Director of the Cassel Hospital. And was from 1997, Professor at the Centre for Psychoanalytic Studies, University of Essex, until 2015.

From 1989, thanks to *Free Association Books* and Bob Young he began an academic interest in psychoanalysis. This led to the publication of the well-known *Dictionary of Kleinian Thought*. This interest has led him to write on many clinical and academic topics, including research on psychiatric and psychoanalytic ethics, on the contributions of psychoanalysis to political thinking, and he has maintained a continuous interest in the application of psychoanalytic ideas to social science. He has also published papers on the history of psychoanalysis, and was jointly responsible with Andrea Sabbadini in stating the Journal *Psychoanalysis and History*.

Despite now being retired from the public service, he is in demand as a speaker and supervisor and travels widely giving talks and workshops, as well as supervising clinicians by skype from his home in Norfolk.

You can see him in action at https://vimeo.com/175839335 and find out about his other writing at www.rdhinshelwood.net

Acknowledgements

I want to thank all those patients of mine who have kept me wondering about my reactions to them. In addition, I am grateful to the many supervisees I have worked with and whose countertransferences they have shown (willingly or unwittingly), which I have tried to be respectful of for the purposes of our joint learning. I have had stimulating discussion on reverie and subjectivity with Josh Holmes. Perhaps I should also thank my own analyst, Stanley Leigh, whose countertransference was always a source of considerable mystery to me, so that it occupied much of my attention and concern. I include gratitude to my own supervisors during my training, Isabel Menzies and Sydney Klein, who were probably as mystified about my countertransferences to my patients as I was. Many colleagues have given support of many kinds, including Wladek Banas; and also people who have been influential in soliciting my earlier publications; Jon Mill, Robert Oelsner, and previous Editors of the IJPA, Glen Gabbard and Paul Williams. I am especially grateful to Em Farrell for pointing the way through the labyrinth of digital, online and conventional publishing. I am also grateful to Nell Norman-Nott for the use of her painting in the cover design.

Preface

As a medical student, during my training on the wards I found it obvious how things worked. Patients were in bed and doctors and nurses bustled around giving near lethal drugs at non-lethal doses, or operating inside sick and unconscious bodies. The passive and the active were clearly defined and played out by these roles. I say "roles" because they were roles rather than persons – or at least, being a person came along second. Each are appreciative of the other, keeping within the roughly defined limits – the patient is a category. Later, it was not a big step for an enquiring mind to come across the literature on the social construction of persons, and I remember reading soon after Berger and Luckmann (1966) *The Social Construction of Reality*, a readily available Penguin paperback.

Then, moving to the psychiatric wards as I did fairly soon after, it was natural to take with me the same role expectations, the same allotted active and passive behaviours required by the designation 'patient'. It was even more prevalent in psychiatry. Active patients were worrying as they were defined as unpredictable, and none could be considered reliable. Psychiatry was a danger zone; patients were incomprehensible. Their passivity could give way to sharp and alarming moments of violent impulsiveness. Their condition could be considered a 'health and safety issue', although that phrase had not yet been invented.

The pressures of these social roles could be irresistible, and vulnerable people needing the benefit of the service took up the positions and behaviour, and indeed identities, given by the frightened staff. At the time, the radical ideas of R.D. Laing (1960) were prominent, and, to a young psychiatrist, inspiring. In no time, I had read the classical work of Isabel Menzies (1960) on the distancing processes that were adopted in nursing practice in a general hospital. How much more so did her findings apply to the distancing processes of psychiatric hospitals? Much later, Rob Barrett (1996) pointed out how psychiatric staff treat illnesses, not patients, which rang bells that echoed thirty years previously in my early days as a trainee psychiatrist.

It was not many years before I took steps away from this role-determined approach to psychiatric patients. In 1969, I began to work in a smallish unit (The Marlborough Day Hospital) where, together with other young staff (Roger Hobdell, Sheena Grunberg, Anna Christian, and Angela Foster amongst many others), we established a therapeutic community; a self-consciously egalitarian mode of thinking that gave patients different roles, and their 'healthy' side was emphasised over their illness and symptoms. At the same time, I began training as a psychoanalyst in the knowledge that there was a glittering tradition in Britain of analysts exploring the experiences and troubles of patients who were psychotic. The therapeutic community was a founding influence, which not only gave a very different view of psychiatry, but also offered a particular perspective on psychoanalysis.

If psychiatry was the impersonal way to help people, then psychoanalysis was supposed to be a much more personal way, listening, empathising with experiences, and being attuned and understanding – understanding both consciously and beyond. In many ways it is all that, but over the years its own history has come to show the origins and limitations of psychoanalysis. There is a sense in which psychoanalysis is used by its practitioners to prove psychoanalysis itself, and especially to prove their own particular theories. Though kindly called analysands, people are used in order to fit symptoms to theories; diagnostic labels are sometimes used as they are in psychiatry; what happens to the analyst is sometimes attributed merely to the patient. Today, the increasing plethora of contesting theories tempts different groups to seek a priority for their theories, so often patients are merely fitted to theories – for the sake of the theories as much as for the patients.

That process is backed by the idealisation of one's own theory, from which it would logically follow that if the theory was so wonderful, then interpretations based on such a theory were bound to be correct ones. That kind of certainty is a considerable comfort for psychoanalysts beset by the uncertainties of the work, and also by the competition and animosity towards each other (Britton and Steiner, 1994; Feldman 2009). A striking degree of objectifying distance can descend on the report of a case in the journals or at conferences. Whilst I can exaggerate this to the point of condemnation, I should not; the situation is infinitely better than the clumsy excesses of the DSM in psychiatry.

I found myself drawn in my work to puzzle over the gathering revolution in the approaches to countertransference, and the place of these certainties, uncertainties and anxieties of the analyst. I encountered psychoanalysis not so long after the seminal papers in 1950 and 1960 by Paula Heimann, the most prominent of the crusaders who were rehabilitating countertransference, and saw its potential usefulness for the understanding of the unconscious communications of the patient.

It has taken me until I have reached touching distance from the end of my career to be able to systematise my thoughts and to write this account. It is composed of the ideas originally appearing in a number of papers on countertransference (Hinshelwood 1997a, 1999a, 2007, 2008, 2009, 2013b) as well as at least an equal number of unpublished papers, written for presentation at various events and occasions.

* * * *

I trained in the Kleinian tradition because the reputation for understanding psychosis, and the experience of those who suffered it, gave considerable respect to Klein's claim that she understood dynamics and unconscious processes at a deeper level than the neurotic level of Oedipus and repression. She was always using the term 'the deeper layers', and it seemed likely that she was on to something. I greatly respected Bion's clarification of the two levels, based on his work with psychosis. He distinguished a psychotic from a non-psychotic part of a personality in the following way:

> The non-psychotic personality was concerned with a neurotic problem, that is to say a problem that centred on the resolution of a conflict of ideas and emotions to which the operation of the ego had given rise. But the psychotic personality was concerned with the problem of repair of the ego (Bion 1957, p. 272)

That is to say, the basic anxiety in psychosis is that the ego will not survive, but will disintegrate in some more or less alarming way. In contrast, an ego that is more secure engages with different anxieties – those of the Oedipus complex and conflicts.

But, that is not the point of this text. The person of the analyst, and his anxieties, is the point. The notion of countertransference embodies the reality that the ego of the analyst struggles too. It is not just that the patient has a transference – the analyst has a countertransference. It is not just that the analyst analyses the patient's personality; the patient gets a very good idea of the analyst's personality (and indeed how he, the patient, might exploit it). It is not just that the analyst is a container for the patient's overflowing feelings, but the patient will contain the analyst almost as much. What a complex entanglement.

If psychoanalysis, like psychiatry, can keep sliding into a technical procedure, 'countertransference' is the great redeeming concept. It must keep in mind that when someone is with a disturbed person, they are both disturbed. It is a simple fact of humanity, and it is a shame we have to use a word that sounds like it is aimed at obfuscation for the uninitiated. In fact, countertransference is the most human of all human characteristics and functions. We relate; we humans do so in a way that nothing else in the universe does. We should be proud of psychoanalysis for creating a fuss about it, even if that includes lots of hot air, and even bad temper. Countertransference is the essence of the live connection between human beings. And, being a property of the precise setting of psychoanalysis, psychoanalysis is therefore the principle means of understanding how relations between people come alive.

Psychoanalysis and its associated dynamic psychotherapies have virtues, unique ones. It is the only psychology to take intimacy seriously. Its uniqueness is not just that it addresses the unconscious mind – it is, of course, unique in that respect as no other psychology takes the unconscious as a field of research and investigation – but it is unique in turning a similar spotlight on intimacy and the humanity of that mutually consuming interest. In this respect, countertransference leads us into the raw difficulties of being human, which interestingly can be turned into an advantage – if only we can see how to turn it that way. This book is about that turning.

* * * *

The instigating moment for this book was coming across Elizabeth Spillius' comment about the rather dry theory-inspired interpretations analysts were often driven to make, and which were likely to have been detrimental to the recognition of alive moments of emotional contact (Spillius, 1988, p. 9). That implicit and unconscious reaction that turns psychoanalysis into a technical procedure has often resulted in the two partners remaining in a distant, only semi-engaged encounter, avoiding the life of a closer relationship. It was many years after musing on hard-to-reach and easy-to-reach patients that I was struck by this remark of Elizabeth Spillius. She was reflecting on this whole area of work concerning the way a patient can employ these concerns of the analyst, and their theories and interpretations, to reduce the session to a defensive operation. Spillius wrote:

> [An analyst] who made interpretations in terms of
> verbal and behavioural content seen in a rigidly symbolic
> form... now seems likely to have been detrimental to
> the recognition of alive moments of emotional contact
> (Spillius, 1988, p. 8-9).

This points to the importance of 'alive moments', and is not so
dissimilar to Freud's thought:

> After all, his [the patient's] conflicts will only be
> successfully solved and his resistances overcome if the
> anticipatory ideas he is given tally with what is real in
> him (Freud, 1917a, p. 452).

This captured my concern to understand the analytic
encounter as a live interaction between two people, and indeed
to understand how it was that a psychoanalysis might go for
long periods with a process that was troublingly lacking in life,
and indeed has been described as nothing short of an impasse
(Rosenfeld, 1987).

Some years after Spillius drew attention to the dead moments
of the stilted pursuit of theory, Ogden acknowledged this also:

> [I had] become increasingly aware over the past several
> years that the sense of aliveness and deadness of the
> transference-countertransference is, for me, perhaps
> the single most important measure of the moment-to-

moment status of analytic process (Ogden, 1995, p. 695).

Though Ogden draws for support from Winnicott (1971), Bion (1959), Symington (1983), Coltart (1986), Green (1983), Bollas (1987), Casement (1985), Meares (1993), Mitchell (1993), and Stewart (1977), Spillius' observation is not there amongst that group dominated by European writers. And there may be a significant reason which can become clearer in Part 2 (Chapters 5, 7 and 8). This is probably because Ogden's approach is different from the approach that Spillius took, and others associated with the work of Betty Joseph (Joseph, 1989) and that of Steiner and of Feldman. The latter concerned themselves with the anxieties of the analyst and the opportunities those anxieties gave patients. For Ogden on the other hand, the aliveness derives more directly from the 'analyst's "realness", i.e. his capacity for spontaneity and freedom... that is not strangulated by stilted caricatures of analytic neutrality' (Ogden, 1995, p. 696). Though there is a similarity in the view of how technique is distorted, there is a difference of emphasis between a more interactive mode, and a focus on personality attributes. These are representative of the two quite divergent views of the countertransference developed in Part 2.

The journey I pursue here with the reader will start with the conventional chronology of the historical and clinical debate, but then emphasise the importance of those moments of life in the clinical process. Those readers who want the kernel of this work must go straight to Part 3, and my account of the use of countertransference today.

Gauging the significance of the alive moments, and the dead ones, is an approach to the analyst's subjectivity as well as the patient's. Our journey includes the importance, over the years, of the problems of intimacy sent to test the helping hand, and it seems to frighten the psychoanalyst as often as not.

The thrilling journey for the analyst, however challenging as well, is the pursuit of alive moments of contact, human to human. These moments are to be treasured.

* * * *

A note on word usage: I have made a decision to use the term 'patient' most often, rather than 'analysand'. There is no good reason for this apart from the fact that 'patient' is common usage, even though it smacks of medicalisation, which I am against; also, referring to the 'analysand' has a slightly pompous quality to it, which I am also against.

More modern terms 'user', or 'expert from lived experience' have struck me as wielding an uncomfortably patronising attitude to those deemed unfortunate. If that were so, then why not stick with the old-fashioned term 'patient' – it does at least, have its common root with 'passive', recognising the human subject as a person who suffers. This book of course is focused on those who 'suffer with' patients, and emphasises how much we are all in the same boat as we are all irredeemably human persons.

Occasionally I shall use the pronoun 'he', 'his', etc., in a generalised ungendered sense, to avoid the cumbersome circumlocutions which might otherwise occur. The specific or the ungendered senses are, I hope, clear from the context each time.

I use the term 'psychoanalysis' in the broadest sense to include the group of psychodynamic therapies which are grounded in one or the other schools of psychoanalytic ideas (Hinshelwood, 2001a). The point is the recognition of the analyst as being emotionally alive in the meeting with his patient, alive to his patient's emotional connection with the analyst, and aware of his own reactions as much as of his technique.

Introduction

In Part 1, I want to cover the historical progress of the idea. As Kierkegaard said, concepts, like people, have biographies. So at the beginning I start with the emotional problem that Jung and Ferenczi posed for Freud and how, in reaction, the psychoanalytic world first set up an objectifying system for controlling the problem, averting a professional contagion. The suspicion then attached to countertransference, reflected how vulnerable our forebears felt and how we are all in intimate contacts and relations with others. That psychoanalytic caution has been long-lasting, and has given rise to a number of pejorative words aimed, it always seems ineffectually, at shaming the analyst via his professional super-ego. Failures at keeping an emotional, hygienic distance have always dogged the psychoanalyst. Nevertheless, a psychoanalyst fails in interesting ways, and Freud's cases were invariably reported for the problems he may have encountered, and then for the ingenious ways he found to understand those errors and to advance the objective truths of psychoanalysis. Theoretical understanding advanced knowledge in general, even if the difficulties hindered the understanding of individuals.

Part 2 is the 'reformation'. The paradigm shift in understanding (and using) countertransference has led to a divergence of views about countertransference, and its synonym, the 'subjectivity' of the analyst. Overall, the emergence of intersubjectivity has marked psychoanalysis in the last 60 years. In particular, the trends separate into two specific ones:

- the intra-psychic; and

- the co-constructivst.

The use of countertransference can be extraordinarily wild, and even Heimann eventually warned of a misuse, a warning that has become more and more important. The capacity to keep to a clinical rigour whilst following one's own feelings has led to difficulties in publicly presenting clinical work, via conferences or publications, in a suitably rigorous way (see Hinshelwood, 2013a for a 'subjective' rigour).

Part 3 is the core of the book, as it reviews the way contemporary thinking embodies countertransference in the clinical setting. I here succumb to a personal preference – the work of Betty Joseph, who prioritised the precise reading of small details of the *process* of the material, the micro-process. This has had enormous ramifications for the development of technique, and also for clinical research, and not only in the Kleinian tradition (see for instance Hanly and Hanly, 2001; Almond 2003; Busch 2015; Eizirik 2010). Joseph's own analysts were firstly Michael Balint during the 1940s, and then Paula Heimann around 1950 or thereabouts; both Balint and Heimann were significant in the re-assessment of countertransference, as Part 2 will try to capture.

Without research results from the clinical setting, we would have no psychoanalytic theory. The frequent doubts expressed (and sometimes trumpeted) about knowledge production from the clinical setting may in part be valid, though the answer is not to abandon that method of gaining our knowledge, but to address the need for greater rigour in using the data of the clinical setting (Hinshelwood, 2013a). The notion of enactment has varying meanings, but generally signifies a diversion from *conscious* knowledge into unconscious active role-playing and relating. Enactments can be, however, the anteroom to a fuller knowledge of human encounters, unconscious especially, as well as conscious. We can even look back at old presentations where the unconscious revealed important insights, if only current knowledge had been available then to read it.

Part 4 then moves cautiously beyond the clinic, to other fields. Caution is required in order not to over-claim for psychoanalytic thinking. The two chapters in this part consider areas where I think it is valid to pursue the importance of the concept of countertransference. First, a brief venture into thoughts about the state and 'health' of contemporary society; and second, the important use of countertransference in research in the clinical setting with the formulation of interpretation and its generalisation.

PART 1

IN HISTORICAL TIMES

Ideas have biographies, too;

> Concepts, like individuals, have their histories and
> are just as incapable of withstanding the ravages of
> time as are individuals. But in and through all this they
> retain a kind of homesickness for the scenes of their
> childhood (Kierkegaard, 1989 [1841] p. 9).

The history of the idea of countertransference is nearly as
long as the history of psychoanalysis itself. In a way they go
together – anxiety and the creative use of countertransference.
Ambivalence towards countertransference has always existed.
However, the ambivalence has tended to separate into two
distinct historical phases; the first, a phase where suspicion and
suppression of countertransference has predominated, and
the second, a phase of revised usage where sometimes, to the
point of idealisation, countertransference has become a major
source of investigative data, albeit data of the subjective kind.

In this Part, the earliest recognition of the phenomenon, and
the alarm generated, is briefly covered.

The particular problem is that the work of psychoanalysts willingly invites the most intimate of intimacies between them and their patients. Analysts unprepared for this assault on their integrity are vulnerable. Perhaps more than a century ago, the paternalism of professions protected practitioners from too much disgrace, which would today be lethal for anyone's career. Chapter 1 shows Freud's complacency over the (male) analyst's complications with their patients (female). So, at the outset Freud faced his colleagues' shame and stood with them. It was a complex enigma since these transgressive acts were in the context of proclaiming psychoanalysis as inherently transgressive, and declaring the unconscious determinants of human experience.

Chapter 2 remarks on the nature of intimacy and the protection from its temptations. Emotional distancing may be the crucial factor in making the alive moments so elusive. Chapter 3 wonders if alive moments can be enabled to survive whilst countertransference remains suffocated by suspicion and prohibition.

CHAPTER 1

Shame amongst friends
What could Freud say?

We will start with the early origins of the suspicion of countertransference; where did it start? The psychoanalyst brings his own inner world of experiences, as well as professional training and knowledge. In a way, this is obvious, but debating it has not been consistently pursued, and spasmodic views on what to do about the analyst's person have appeared from time to time, some gaining dominance for a while, and others sinking to oblivion in the discarded literature.

That the analyst must indeed struggle – at least consciously – with his own reactions to the patient has made countertransference a significant paradox for clinical psychoanalysis. Whilst those reactions are unconscious ones, we can only struggle consciously. So, facing countertransference full in the face is not straightforward, especially as it has to be done on a constant basis. Psychoanalysis is not like other professions; it is the profession that dwells on the problems of the very practice of a profession. It is known that lawyers, for instance, are unfortunately prone to step aside from proper conduct and engage in sympathetic intimacy, especially with their divorcing clients. Psychoanalysts, exposed to the same risk, are not only required to abstain, but are also required to explore such feelings as countertransference.

So, do the psychoanalyst's feelings, when working with patients' feelings, interfere? And if they do, could the interference be helpful? Freud was not altogether consistent. On one hand he said, 'he must turn his own unconscious like a receptive organ towards the transmitting unconscious of the patient' (Freud, 1912, p. 115), as if the psychoanalyst's professional contact must be of that ultimately intimate degree.

At the same time, we know Freud was very wary of countertransference. First of all, his suspicion was aroused in the early days when Jung and others had problems, and found themselves in compromising situations with patients, Freud was confronted with these as a serious difficulty. Jung and Ferenczi confided in Freud. They both had overwhelming feelings towards female patients, acted out in the case of Jung (Carotenuto, 1982).

Jung conducted an analysis of Sabina Spielrein from 1905-1909, at which point Spielrein then contacted Freud for a further analysis in Vienna. She, eventually, with Freud's blessing, joined the psychoanalytic profession in 1911. However, in 1909 when Speilrein wrote to Freud, she asked for some unspecified help, and for a brief audience; 'It has to do with something of greatest importance to me which you would probably be interested to hear about' (Letter Spielrein to Freud, 30th May 1909; Carotenuto, 1984, p. 91). This was before Jung and Freud made their fateful trip to the US together (September 1909). So, Freud wrote to Jung in tones somewhat disparaging of the patient, 'What is she? A busybody, a chatterbox, or a paranoic?' (Letter Freud to Jung, 3rd June 1909; McGuire, 1974, p, 169). Jung responded immediately, though in a somewhat similar vein:

> Since I knew from experience that she would immediately relapse if I withdrew my support, I prolonged the relationship over the years and in the end found myself morally obliged, as it were, to devote a large measure of friendship to her, until I saw that an unintended wheel had started turning, whereupon I finally broke with her. She was, of course, systematically planning my seduction, which I considered inopportune. Now she is seeking revenge. Lately she has been spreading a rumour that I shall soon get a divorce from my wife and marry a certain girl student, which has thrown not a few of my colleagues into a flutter. What she is now planning is unknown to me. Nothing good, I suspect, unless perhaps you are imposed upon to act as a go-between. I need hardly say that I have made a clean

break (Letter Jung to Freud, 4th June 1909; McGuire 1974, p. 228-229).

Freud's reaction was remarkably reassuring, saying:

> I myself have never been taken in quite so badly, but I have come very close to it a number of times and had a narrow escape. I believe that only grim necessities weighing on my work, and the fact that I was ten years older than yourself when I came to ΨA, have saved me from similar experiences. But no lasting harm is done. They help us to develop the thick skin we need and to dominate "countertransference,"... They are a "blessing in disguise." (Letter Freud to Jung, 7th June 1909; McGuire, 1974, p. 230-231).

He came to the un-psychoanalytic conclusion that analysts should 'suppress' their feelings. The recommendation to Jung is a conscious one – to develop a thick skin, and to dominate the countertransference. This is surprising since he was also telling the world about the strength of the *unconscious* determinants beyond conscious control.

A few years later, in a letter completed on January 31st 1912, Ferenczi described his complex affection for both Frau G (Gisella Pallos) and her daughter Elma. Elma was in analysis with Ferenczi, and Ferenczi had fallen in love with her. He also had a close relationship with Gisella (who had previously had a brief analysis with Ferenczi, and whom he later married), about whom Ferenczi said at this point, 'She wanted to remain completely on the ground of the sublimated' (Letter Ferenczi to Freud, 31st January 1912; Brabant et al., 1993, p. 336). He continued:

> [B]ut I (in order to flee Elma) pressed for a resumption of the old relation. It did *not go well*. It was becoming more and more apparent that I haven't entirely given Elma up and that at least a part of my sexual desires [towards Giesella] were not genuine. My attempt at intimacy ended with sadness and depression on both sides (Letter Ferenczi to Freud, 28th/31st January 1912; Brabant et al., 1993, p. 336).

Freud replied immediately on February 1st, expressing respect for Ferenczi's confidence, and responding:

> What you report to me about the changes in your relationship with Frau G. was not surprising at all. I had presumed that it would go first one way and then the other. There is nothing to be ashamed of in that, even though it is not right (Freud 1912b, [Letter Freud to Ferenczi, 1st February 1912; Brabant et al., 1993, p. 340).

Freud was again reassuring and tolerant. Though he recognised the shame, for Ferenczi's sake he denied it (even though, as he said, it is not right).

Freud needed his colleagues at the time, and was duly supportive. Despite Freud's apparent complacency in his correspondence, these manifestations of countertransference gave rise to the classical view that countertransference is a pathological manifestation in the analyst stimulated by the patient's transference. Freud recommended adopting the steely attitude of assumed neutrality characteristic of 'a surgeon, who puts aside all his feelings, even his human sympathy, and concentrates his mental forces on the single aim of performing the operation as skilfully as possible' (Freud, 1912, p, 115). By the 1920s, the eventual consequence of this view of countertransference as the analyst's disturbance was that all new psychoanalysts should undergo their own analysis, in order that they might put aside their feelings and sympathy.

Freud was puzzled by the non-verbal process of unconscious-to-unconscious communication from which these untoward and unethical occurrences emerged, and unclear what actual mechanisms could bring them about. Ferenczi, it seems, even persuaded Freud to go to a spiritualist séance to study the possibility of thought transmission directly from one mind to another without going through the cognitive and verbal channels of communication. Freud, it seems, was unimpressed with such thought transmission and remained puzzled (see Letter Freud to Ferenczi, 23rd November 1913; Brabant et al., 1993).

So disturbances in the analyst began to emerge early on as a specific concern. Glover devoted the fourth of his lectures on technique in psychoanalysis in 1927 to a specific investigation of countertransference. He began to think of the way the analyst relates to the patient's emotional state: 'We might almost say, "When in difficulty think of your own repressed sadism"' (Glover, 1927, p. 510).

Ferenczi, on the other hand, always pushed for more intimacy. His letters to Freud were always personal and invited the return, to the point where one might consider him disappointed by Freud. Eventually, in the 1920s, Ferenczi proceeded to develop his professional relationship with Groddeck in more personal ways, and they set up a mutual analysis (Dupont, 1988). After Michael Balint translated Ferenczi's *Clinical Diary* in 1988, Ferenczi's character became open to discussion:

> Ferenczi wanted Freud to be both his analyst and a participant in his life, a contradictory combination of roles. However, since the small community of early analysts repeatedly attempted to overcome this identical dilemma with one another, it is not surprising

that Ferenczi should be confused and that his analysis would be interminable (Ginsberg, 1991, p. 295).

Ferenczi's work has become much better known in the last 25 years or so. His brave experiments – such as his attempts at mutual analysis with patients (Dupont, 1988) – were not mainstream psychoanalysis at the time, and are not now. They are important as a divergent strand from the rather sterner orthodoxy that the mainstream psychoanalysts promoted. Ferenczi's adventurous explorations of countertransference did not coincide with the 'official' suspicion, and probably contributed to the cooling of relations between him and Freud in the 1920s. We now know much more about Ferenczi's experiments with intimacy in his clinical practice with his patients. Not just being enamoured with his patient Elma and her mother Gisella, but experimenting with something like a mutual analysis by swapping places on the couch. These experiments, whilst not condoned, have nevertheless retained an impact, and led to more measured and thoughtful experiments which retain the analyst's humanity rather than burying it behind the surgeon's scalpel wielded upon an unconscious body.

CHAPTER 2

Distantiation, said Erikson
What could they all do?

Psychoanalysis places considerable stresses on the practitioner, as do all caring and professional occupations. The expectation is that the professional will conduct himself impeccably in an emotionally neutral way; as the American humourist, Ogden Nash, for instance, quipped:

> Professional men, they have no cares
> Whatever happens, they get theirs

> (Ogden Nash, 1935)

However, for the analyst grappling with the unconscious forces, elements of his fellow-feeling with his patient are especially obscure, hidden and intimate. The effects of those unconscious pressures are difficult to manage and use. Instead, their threat may be dealt with by condemning, suppressing, indulging in, or analysing away, and thus ape Nash's humorous caricature.

The word 'intimacy' is sometimes used as a coy synonym for penetrative sexuality (at least in English), though not always, of course. In that bodily sense, it may indicate the importance of closeness, but including the possibility that it can become an inappropriate over-involvement, an intrusive, even violating, closeness. It has always been a problem for psychoanalysts who aim to discuss the most intimate secrets of one person, whilst retaining a professional attitude, i.e. a step back from a personal involvement. Over the years, analysts' protection has been to distance themselves from their own emotional contact with the patient, with the forms of objectification described.

Intimacy and its conflicts

Now, why has intimacy required such a protective shield? All professions are about the personal affairs of the client, so intimacy in professional life seems a particular threat. The reactions are inevitably varied, and often desperate. The troubled clients of mental health professionals are particularly solicitous of more intimate care than is professionally appropriate. Psychoanalysts are the professionals most likely to be challenged. Their work is especially intimate, and at the same time they are the people expected to know most about the conflicts over intimate contact.

The term 'intimacy' is not a technical term in psychoanalysis, although Erikson employed a simple definition – to 'lose oneself in the meeting of bodies and minds' (Erikson, 1950, p. 231); this sparks off a plethora of resonances for psychoanalysts. It seems it may not just be a respect for the strictures of professional ethics, but also the even more painful problem of losing oneself, a sense of losing one's identity in the role a patient unconsciously demands.

It is a baby's fate to start life with the job of marking the distinction between itself and mother – both in body and in mind. However, a merging may also be profoundly longed for, for various reasons. It is a highly conflicted state of being with others – close yet distinct. This warns of the twin problems, the Scylla and Charybdis, of the countertransference – emotionally freezing like the steely surgeon; or being over-human and seduced out of role – ultimately, perhaps, into unethical relations, and even towards problems of self and identity. The analyst is required to pay attention to this intimate linking, or 'mating', as Brenman Pick called it. Disentangling this entanglement is the process she named 'working through in the countertransference' (Brenman Pick, 1985).

That inherent conflict from the outset of our lives, and its colouring of all the phases of our development, is something that psychoanalysts are not immune from. Moreover, the nature of our work brings us up against the conflict in a way that is foreign to other professions. Whilst perhaps most other caring professions may simply repudiate that intensity of meeting (see Menzies, 1959), psychoanalysts have to know that intimacy, in its earliest forms, it is the nature of our work. Because of our especial closeness in the work, i.e. an intimacy with the subjective experiencing of others, it would be surprising if these conflicts were *not* significant for us. One American analyst went so far as to say, more than 50 years ago:

> For some persons the problem of intimacy is the principal determinant of the vocational choice of psycho-analysis (Wheelis, 1956, p. 180).

The problem of intimacy is that it threatens the experience of being a person. The closeness between self and the other person risks obliterating the boundary altogether. Erikson (1950), somewhat surprisingly, dates this conflict to young adulthood. However there is no reason to follow that paradigm when dissolution of the self appears to be a very primitive anxiety, and therefore one that might be found from very early in development. What Erikson described with some empirical grounds is that the conflict, however early it starts, is a determinant of adult life as well.

Erikson argued that distance is the typical, protective response to the threat of intimacy:

> The counterpart of intimacy is distantiation: the readiness to isolate and, if necessary, to destroy those forces and people whose essence seems dangerous to one's own, and whose 'territory' seems to encroach on

the extent of one's intimate relations (Erikson, 1965 [1950], p. 255).

In other words, the reaction to the threat of intimacy and loss of self is to move away, and create an emotionally suppressed or deadened process.

We might conclude that the thick-skinned suppression of the emotional countertransference contact would appear to be not just a proper regard for professional conduct, but a method of self-protection. This factor goes beyond professional conduct, and this fundamental human anxiety might well be a hidden factor that we have not yet addressed as a profession.

We might briefly consider this further. Psychoanalysts move so readily into dispute and debate that it is a big issue for psychoanalysis and its warring institutions (see for instance Kirsner, 1999). Of course, any discipline is alive with debate. Once debate and controversy disappear, then the discipline has died, as it no longer has the wherewithal to sustain progress. There are real issues of theory and debate to be discussed, investigated and resolved. What is critical in the psychoanalytic world is the lack of resolution. The preference, it almost seems, is to live with unresolvable differences between colleagues. When such mysterious preferences are evident, and not amenable to ordinary debate, there is a fair enough suspicion that they depend on unconscious factors—and this may occur even amongst analysts. The debates about countertransference over the last century may constitute one such unconscious factor. It is a hidden conflict, and it is not resolved precisely because it is hidden. I suggest that one hidden driver of such endless debate arises from the difficulty in all human beings to sustain intimacy with others in general. Countertransference in particular is a pressure to relinquish the professional stance.

The core question of this chapter – what is to be done? – requires these issues to be explored. However, in some respects, the fear of intimacy and human responsiveness has led to the intensification of and the narrowing of the focus onto the patient's psychology and psychopathology:

> A cursory glance at the syllabus of any representative body of psychologists is sufficient to remind us how rarely psychotherapists inflict on themselves the discipline of self-examination. Papers on the subject matter of clinical investigation are as plentiful as blackberries, but only once in a while is the instrument of investigation, the psychotherapist himself, subjected to purposive scrutiny (Glover, 1928, p. 1).

The threatening experience a countertransference may provoke, is in fact an authentic human contact. It may be suppressed for its unconscious threat; however, it could also be sentimentally idealised as especially human. Both would be defensive reactions.

Some strategies

Psychoanalysts typically learn an approach to their countertransference feelings in the course of their training, not least from the attitude of their own analyst.

Using pejorative words: In the early days, the unconscious pressures of countertransference were a threat that became expressed as a negative assessment and attracted the use of pejorative descriptions. Over the years, almost knee-jerk responses to countertransference have given rise to a condemning vocabulary as a seemingly rather desperate means of dealing with the risk of unprofessional intimacy. Those methods of attempting to suppress intimate feelings have led to terms carrying various degrees of criticism, and it has sustained a distance against the suspected threat of countertransference for near on a century.

The term 'collusion' was introduced in the 1920s, indicating the subversive influence between the unconscious of two persons. From the 1930s, the term 'acting-out' came into use, and similarly represented an implicit criticism that what should be restricted to words and the transference relationship in the session, had leaked into relations outside the analysis. It was disapproved of because it impoverished the analytic process within the session, but the idea of the *analyst* acting-out with the patient became prominent later (in the 1950s) as a serious lapse. That amounted to an 'enactment' which, originally more or less synonymous with the *patient* acting-out, and comparable to what Freud in 1912 called repeating, has come more into use.

Other related terms euphemistically indicating psychoanalytic failures – 'impasse', 'stuckness', 'negative therapeutic reaction' – represent in many instances a slippage from the task of learning, and so imply a shameful loss of emotional neutrality,

Freud's recommendations on technique thoroughly explored transference as an *active* repetition of a trauma or a relationship, in contrast to a remembrance that could be put into words (Freud, 1915). The original conflict or trauma is re-enacted as the transference relationship. The analyst should refrain from acting-out with the patient. However, this unconscious drama reaches beyond the 'should', and may be enacted by both parties in a transference-countertransference interaction. Both are drawn into the drama, the analyst is sometimes drawn by the patient, sometimes by his own unconscious.

This places words in a key position. That focus, to some extent, corroborated Freud's very early neurological work on aphasia (Freud, 1891, 1915), and countertransference emphasised further the need for the talking cure to be restricted to talking. Only words and not actions, not even emotional responses, were permissible; anything else was a resistance to be interpreted by the analyst for the purposes of verbal insight.

This reliance on words was reinforced by the sense that the analyst all too frequently, like the patient, can unconsciously enact instead of verbalise. Such terms imply a degree of disapproval at the insightlessness, and they diverge from the analogy of Freud's steely surgeon. The development of these pejorative descriptions suggests that despite the introduction of a training analysis in the 1920s, analysts unwittingly continued to allow reprehensible phenomena deriving from the countertransference to occur. Such phenomena were to be identified in the supervision of trainees and new analysts (via their 'control' analyses), but also became a currency for critical appraisal of each other.

The blank screen: It is clear that the functioning of the analyst's personality, his own subjectivity and his unconscious, has never been a settled issue. The list of damning words that the analyst's super-ego could throw at himself – or at other analysts – represents a fear of the potential over-whelming involvement, an overwhelming *unconscious* involvement. So, countertransference has been persistently fretted over, and has generated this emotionally toned vocabulary to assist analysts in protecting themselves by keeping a distance from emotional contact. However, in the actual setting the distantiation has taken the form of the blank screen, which doubles as a thick skin so that the patient's transferred drama is projected as if in the cinema. But, the countertransference feelings – and enactments did not subside with a policy of name-calling.

The terms suggest that the professional responsibility was to remain steely. The 'blank screen' as it came to be called by Jelliffe (1930), commenting on James Glover (1926), expressed the analyst's continuing conflict over going along with the patient in this intimate way. Terese Benedek (1953) summed up the position: 'As the history of psychoanalysis shows, the discussion of countertransference usually ended in a retreat to defensive positions' (Benedek, 1953, p. 202).

That retreat has been the expression, in the technical form of correct procedure, of Freud's early recommendation for a conscious suppression and the adoption of the thick skin. Onto this thick skin, as if a cinema screen, the patient is allowed to project a narrative of primitive roles that have cluttered and determined his/her unconscious processing of experience, with the production of symptoms rather than sublimations. The blank screen is potentially a device for 'seeing' the unconscious in dramatic form, as if played out in a theatre, a cinema or a play room.

These criticisms over the years were documented by Hoffman (1983). The concern seems to have been expressed in the safe arena of journals and books. However, when it has come to the practice in the actual clinical setting, there has been a tendency to retreat behind this screen.

Abstracting intimacy: The need to capture the process in a strongly terminological framework unfortunately reduces the human process of relating and intimacy to a deadening formal conceptualisation. As if, having captured the wild animal in this verbal and conceptual cage, maybe its danger would be tamed. But, as we introduce those abstractions for emotional relating, however relevant, we have made a move towards distancing and losing touch with the risk and benefits of the emotional (and often erotic) grounding in experience. The abstractions have assisted in creating the emotional distance. Even those most committed to the authenticity of each partner's subjectivity can become involved in abstract debate (*about* authenticity perhaps). As such, the authentic experiencing has been pushed into the distance.

Freud thought the unconscious nature of the process could be overcome when over-arching theory could be relied upon to shape the process. With the plethora of psychoanalytic theories, it is no longer possible to apply a theory as if it is a universally accepted feature of the unconscious. Analysts have a whole storehouse of theories available to them. Moreover, as Sandler (1983) said, analysts have 'implicit theories' as well (see Tuckett et al., 2008). As a consequence, analysts will be tempted to 'read' their countertransference in many different ways, and match it in accord with theory more than with personal perspectives. Theory is nicely impersonal, as it removes the threat of intimacy. However, gambits with concepts are no less defensive than an onslaught of pejorative epithets, or the thick skin screening out of the emotional narrative.

CHAPTER 3

Wanted dead or alive
What are live moments?

Much of the visibility of countertransference can be covered by the use of pejorative condemnation, or the distancing practice of the blank screen. Especially in the clinical encounter, the lively engagement may be avoided by abstract conjecture that deadens the intimate process. These implicit and unconscious reactions allow the setting to become one in which the two partners remain in a distant, only semi-engaged, contact, avoiding the liveliness of a closer relatedness. Spillius' description (of the importance of alive moments) implied that the opposite, a characteristic deadness, occurs in its place.

I exemplify this with one mid-week session of a middle-aged man, who was difficult to engage with, and in fact occasionally went literally to sleep during sessions. Only infrequently could we get a sense of engagement together:

> He told me of a meeting he had with a friend with whom he was working on a project. The friend did very little towards the project, rarely contributed what

he had agreed to do, and was in fact a very unreliable man. However my patient was extraordinarily fond of and loyal to this friend. On this occasion I found myself thinking what an unreliable patient I had, who at times would literally go to sleep on the project I was conducting with him. I felt a mixture of irritation that I was struggling so much to make headway with his analysis. I interpreted this a little mechanically along these lines. I compared how we both struggled to keep a project going, him with his friend, and I with him. He was silent (in fact a common response for him), and then he started snoring (also common).

There is no sign of an alive moment in that... There was, on my part, a mechanical interpretation of verbal content. The interpretation had the quality of what one of my supervisors, long before when I was training, told me was a 'you-mean-me' transference interpretation – the mechanical quality of translating the content of the associations onto the alternative figure of the analyst.

The question would be: What happened to the analyst that he used a mechanical mode of thinking? He too was not 'alive', and contributed his share of the deadness to the moment. In the actual session, the process seemed aimed at moving away from this alive irritation. This entailed taking the content and substituting different figures into the narrative described, just as Freud had done 100 years before in his thematic analysis of his dreams. It points strongly towards the fact that a simple content analysis is in fact too simple. What is the missing ingredient?

The deadness appears to be the analyst's responsibility, but what prompted him to go in this incorrect direction? The analyst was irritated, and, in my description, conveyed a sense of hopelessness with this man. It might be supposed I think, that, with charity, the analyst did his best to just keep going— and what that meant was that he avoided the irritation. In that moment, perhaps irritation was the missing liveliness (see Chapter 15 for a further instalment of this vignette).

When Freud translated his dream interpretation method to the clinical situation with Dora (in 1899), he too employed a version of the you-mean-me transposition. In that work, Freud transposed elements of the dream meaning. What he also neglected was that there was a real live issue right there with him and Dora in the session. He failed to realise that he was regarded as Herr K (Dora's seducer), in what seemed perhaps a powerful and painful manner that impelled Dora to leave. All he could subsequently say was that:

> [There was] some detail in our relations, or in my person or circumstances, behind which there lay

concealed something analogous but immeasurably more important concerning Herr K (Freud, 1905, pp. 118-119).

Freud is conveying a fit between an aspect of transference, and the analyst onto whom it is transferred (at least as perceived by Dora). There was an 'unknown quantity in me', and so she enacted her revenge and deserted Freud for his similar exploitation that seemed to correspond with Herr K's. For Dora, one can see that Freud's dogged work over session after session to work on the dream might not have brought the relevant *relationship* to light. Maybe Herr K's (attempted) seduction of Dora was a mechanical approach too. We don't know what Dora made of Freud, which prodded her to flee the analysis. However, we can say with some certainty that Freud did not allow the relationship to come to life, and the persistent dream symbol interpretation was probably deadening for the adolescent girl. The interpretation of symbols may perhaps tend to be deadening in certain ways for certain people. It suggests that something more than a decoding approach is needed.

Writing a full-length text is evidence of the complexity of the issues provoked by the humanity of the psychoanalyst in the form of countertransference. So often, the difficulties that crop up in an analysis are left simply with the patient; the problem gets reduced simplistically to

– He did it to me...

– A co-production…

– I feel he/she is...

What is not so easily focused on is: What of me did he do it to? That was what Freud, at last, asked in the Dora case, though was not with hindsight able to answer clearly.

It was many years after musing on hard-to-reach (and easy-to-reach) patients that I was struck by Elizabeth Spillius' remark that I mentioned early on. Spillius was reflecting on this whole area of work that Betty Joseph (1989) had opened up, concerning the way a patient can employ the analyst, and the analyst's theories and interpretations, so that together they reduce the session to a defensive operation and stifle live moments.

When the experience does liven up, what is it that comes alive?

Alive moments

Alive moments can be strongly suggestive of when the beginning of an engagement with something really disturbing is on the horizon. When a patient is reached, a moment of life erupts in the session, because his point of suffering has, at last, begun to make a visible entrance.

Prior to the Dora case, Freud had thought of transference as a reservoir of positive affect to be deployed by the analyst, like a military general deploying his troops for battle. The transference became the co-operative element in the patient. The analyst gathered that force to storm the repression; he wielded the power to enable more of the unconscious to emerge into the free associations and dreams. But Dora confounded that. She developed a *negative* transference. It arose from that characteristic in Freud that resembled Herr K, and which aroused Dora's anger or frustration. So while Freud related to the two dreams, Dora related to the analyst. And perhaps there was something of Herr K's seductiveness which Dora thought she saw (or perhaps it was really there) in Freud. We have to presume that Freud did not see Dora's elicit excitement and self-protective terror. Also very speculatively, possibly such an erotic fascination in Freud's countertransference did arouse this young girl. So, Freud then reacted with his exclusive intellectual concentration on the dreams—his form of distancing from the live emotion into intellectual work. And possibly, Freud's actual exploitation (using Dora to evolve his precious theories) was already apparent unconsciously in Freud's interest in her, which became sexual for Dora.

Landmarks

We need guidance and landmarks in order to find our way

in our practice. For the long first phase in the history of psychoanalysis, the guiding principle was to interpret the symbolic coding of experience as it occurred in dreams, symptoms and free associations, and then to find patterns that pointed to general theories, in particular Oedipal conflicts. Then, the process of unfolding in the session becomes calm and emotionally orderly with sensible discussion *about* problems, conflicts, anxieties, defences, dynamics, etc. In fact, such a comfortable capacity for discussion may be a relief, and sought by the patient – and analyst. However, as we have seen it is in itself a move away from something the patient brings that is very disturbing, and towards something that looks like a sophisticated psychoanalytic understanding. It is one of the well-known pitfalls to which the analytic process is vulnerable, in which the patient is greatly relieved by the analyst using a discourse about disturbance in order to protect the patient from feeling it (in fact, to protect both parties). Patients who are especially good at this are then indeed 'hard to reach' (Joseph, 1975).

Dead moments are the indicators of a particular unconscious role the analyst has entered into, which ensure co-operation with the patient in a particular defensive process – very often, as just discussed, this process can be the mechanical interpretation of symbolic contents and meanings. Despite Freud's discovery of the meaning of dream symbols, an overemphasis on simplistic symbol interpretation becomes deadening and defeating – an event that Freud himself recognised in his self-disparaging claim that a cigar is not always a phallic object, sometimes it is only a cigar.

Conclusion

Subsequently, especially after Freud's death in 1939, new generalised theories began to flourish and created a fertile, though unruly, kind of undergrowth. A new factor came into play. Waiting in the wings at the time of Freud's death were other intimations. Instead of the analyst, like a doctor, assigning patients to diagnostic categories, he plays more of a part in relation to the patient. This new factor suggested paying more attention to process in the session (Balint and Balint, 1939, see Chapter 4), and less to the patient's personality structure and content of his communication. It is a difference perhaps of emphasis, but an important difference nonetheless. It pointed toward the 'action' in the here-and-now; the awareness of 'doing things with words'[1]. The 'doing' is of course an unconscious 'doing', the repeating that Freud emphasised (Freud, 1914), and now we understand it as the enacting that draws the analyst into responding to the patient's dramas.

This has implied a change in the old view of transference, which

---

1 The phrase 'doing things with words' comes from the philosopher, J.L. Austin 1962, and a similar idea is conveyed with the notion of non-verbal communication.

was simply the placing of a role on the non-resisting analyst. It means that the so-called 'blank screen' of the analyst should not be so blank, and could activate a process that Sandler eventually termed the 'role responsiveness' of the analyst (Sandler, 1976), or role-actualisation (Sandler, 1993). The analyst (no longer merely a screen) would then allow the performance of that interactive role-playing type of process, in order that it might be recognised and followed, viewed, exposed and understood. However, there is the risk that in the process of playing a role (consciously or unconscious), the analyst is likely to be moved, and thus in danger. Coming alive in the role means something like an engagement, a personal connection and relationship, however unconsciously that might be set up. It should not be seen as acting a drama in the sense of theatre, not a simulation of affects in a role, but as the analyst being genuinely moved to authentic emotional experiences that occupy his attention.

Alive moments are dangerous if not captured in the analyst's conscious understanding, and dead moments are not merely dead, but devotedly ranged against that understanding. More of this complex entanglement in the contemporary clinical use of countertransference can be found in Part 3 of this book. First, the historical moment of transition.

PART TWO

PARADIGM SHIFT

Although the first generation of psychoanalysts tended to condemn and suppress countertransference, there was always a different estimation lurking in the shadows. The dominant trend, to condemn, did not completely snuff out the other interest, the potential for intimacy. In this part, we shall consider how intimacy came out of the shadows and this secondary, submerged view slowly emerged to become the new dominant trend.

During the 1930s, there was truly a psychoanalytic disaster on the European continent, as

Society after Society was eradicated by the political tide of fascism. This was happening at the same time that Freud died, in 1939. The British Society was the one significant European Society left, and it had perforce to contain all this. At this particularly difficult juncture, survival of psychoanalysis itself was the key issue. It was from that apocalyptic epoch that countertransference emerged in the renewed form. The British Society – with its emphasis on the relations with objects – was the one Society that was most likely to give sympathetic attention to the new countertransference.

The transition circa 1950 – from countertransference as bad, to countertransference as good – was not such a clear-cut change. Rather, there have always been two contrasting views, each stemming from Freud. One of them became dominant at first – countertransference as a threat to objectivity and professionalism. This attitude lasted for four or more decades, and the formalism of psychoanalysis in the US retained this more depersonalised view of countertransference even longer[2], although there was also an undercurrent in the US that eschewed the blank screen surgical approach in practice. Perhaps Harold Searles especially represented that resistance; and Erich Fromm published his book, *The Crisis of Psychoanalysis* in 1970. Even where there had been a formal allegiance to the thick-skinned recommendation for suppression of the analyst's feelings, there was a *sotto voce* contrasting appeal to the more personal qualities of the analytic interaction.

So, the transition was not a sudden recognition of countertransference as a useful instrument, rather the submerged view began to resurface.

The paradigm shift now embraced a view of countertransference as the total of *all* the psychoanalyst's feelings arising in the

2   When Bion addressed audiences in America, in 1967, on the interference that memories and desires introduce into the listening process, he was greeted with incomprehension and bewilderment – see Appendix to Aguayo and Malin 2013).

context with a specific patient. It is sometimes called the wider view of countertransference, and it moves much closer to a fuller human encounter between two people. It is a distinct move away from the psychoanalyst as *merely* a trained and knowledgeable professional.

Before surveying in detail one contemporary method of conceiving and using countertransference clinically, the final chapter of Part 2 is a kind of interlude, Chapter 9, where we will look backwards. If the existence of countertransference as an informative interaction between psychoanalyst and patient can be seen in the days *before* that clinical conception had been formulated, then it could be said to have some validity. This represents a small experiment on the textual data we have available. We can test the validity of the wider countertransference as potentially informing the unsuspecting material from the past.

CHAPTER 4

Ferenczi and British psychoanalysis
What put British psychoanalysis ahead?

Alongside Freud's thick-skin approach to countertransference, the non-dominant tradition had survived in the form of Ferenczi's experiments. In the US, the criticisms Searles and Fromm made of mechanistic psychoanalysis reflected a similar trend. Sullivan had also developed his original interpersonal theory that stressed the whole relational field (Sullivan, 1953; Conci, 2010). That interpersonal perspective was not a view congenial to Freud, so the 'native American' tradition struggled to survive the inflow of orthodox psychoanalysts from Vienna and Germany in the 1930s (Kirsner, 1999).

Ferenczi's insistence on a human and mutual relationship with his patients was not always easy, and was possibly even unethical (for instance, the involved passions of the situation with Elma and Gisella Pallos). The long-standing variation that Ferenczi represented (Haynal, 1998) endured after him, especially in the work of Alice and Michael Balint in Budapest, and then in Britain when they took refuge there in 1938.

The non-dominant tradition

Ferenczi had conceived of a field of interaction (Haynal, 1999; and the Barangers, 2008), and Balint followed in this tradition[3]. Fifteen years after Ferenczi died, Balint summarised thus:

> [T]he analytical situation is the result of an interplay between the patient's transference and the analyst's counter-transference, complicated by the reactions released *in each by the other's transference* on to him. (Balint and Balint, 1939, p. 228; italics added)

By this time, the Balints had emigrated to Britain. The political turbulence across Europe after 1914 – not only World War 1, but the Bolshevik Revolution, the Great Depression, the rise of lethal racial supremacy, and World War 2 – led to the very considerable migrations that changed the geography of psychoanalysis. European psychoanalysis was more or less reduced to the British Psychoanalytical Society from the late-1930s; and Russian psychoanalysis had petered out under Stalin. Only small Societies in Switzerland and Sweden survived during the Nazi conquests. The unplanned mixing of different traditions led to controversies over ideas and practice (King and Steiner, 1991; Kirsner, 1999) with largely unresolved and unsatisfactory conclusions.

---

3   Michael and Alice Balint were both analysed in Vienna by Hans Sachs, and Michael Balint subsequently had an analysis in Budapest with Ferenczi.

Alice and Michael Balint brought Ferenczi's influence to Britain in the late 1930s, and their views foreshadowed a trend over the next decade to review the characteristics and importance of countertransference, leading to the seminal paper by Paula Heimann in 1950.

The Viennese influx into the US led to the continuing dominance there of the thick-skin strategy. The suspicious view of countertransference had given strength to the later development of ego psychology and its emphasis on a deterministic, and even mechanistic, objectivity about the vicissitudes of the drives, from the 1930s. However, pockets of the non-dominant tradition remained, deriving in part from the Sullivan tradition augmented by Searles, Horney and Fromm.

In Britain, the situation was more complex. Already, there had been differences between London and Vienna (see the Exchange Lectures – Jones, 1935; Riviere, 1936; Waelder, 1937). As well as Sandor Ferenczi (Ernest Jones, and John Rickman were both analysands of Ferenczi), there were also contacts with Karl Abraham, who represented the first steps towards an object-relations approach, which became much later a distinctive feature of British psychoanalysis. A number of analysts received their analysis from Abraham in Berlin; the two brothers, James and Edward Glover, and Alix

Srachey, wife of James Strachey. These were influential people in London. Hans Sachs moved to Berlin in 1920 (previously part of Freud's Wednesday Group), and there he analysed Ella Freeman Sharpe, and Nina Searl. What these British analysts brought back from Berlin seems to have formed a climate of emerging ideas that enabled Melanie Klein to feel at home when she arrived in 1926.

Abraham had been taking the first cautious steps towards an object-relations view such that the object is more than the passive instrument of the ego's satisfaction. The object is endowed with mental attributes and loved for itself, so not merely for the drive satisfactions it provides – 'whole object love', Abraham called it. It has its own intentions and is loved precisely because it is felt to want to give the satisfactions it provides (or at the opposite pole, the object is hated because it desires the frustrations and pain it is felt to cause). This means that if these ideas were extended to the transference setting, the relationship with the 'object', the analyst, would be conceived very differently. The object would be seen as having a mind of its own and not passively available for satisfaction, or lack of it. These ideas were only modestly conveyed by Abraham, and he did not discuss technique or the countertransference. It seems likely, however, that this almost implicit divergence was picked up by the British psychoanalysts who went to Berlin for their analysis with Abraham.

Melanie Klein was analysed by both Ferenczi and Abraham, and would have found a lot of compatriot camaraderie in London. Ferenczi's tradition, transported to Britain by the Balints in the late 1930s, found a long tradition of psychoanalysis that had been directed towards an emphasis on the object, and object-relations, rather than psychic economics and drive theory. The British Society, long before the diaspora from Vienna, had various incipient influences.

Whilst Abraham and Ferenczi were very different analysts with different ideas and forms of practice, their ideas could both diverge from the standard theories, one in terms of handling intimacy (Ferrenczi), and the other in terms of the felt nature of the object.

The revolution

The growth of revisionism over countertransference was therefore fairly natural once the ego-psychologists in Vienna had been eradicated by the Nazi Anschluss in 1938, and moved largely to the US (although a small but significant group of them, including Anna Freud, remained in London). The blank-screen view of the analyst's role began to come under an increasingly penetrating critique from all schools, for example, Alice Balint (1936) in Budapest, and Fenichel (1941).

The Balints, now in Britain, became a part of a tradition that was not so hostile to underlying ideas about objects, from which the wider view of countertransference arose (e.g. Glover, 1927). During the 1940s, several people were reconsidering countertransference: Milner (1953), Winnicott (1949), Heimann, then a core member of Klein's increasingly embattled group, and further afield, Racker (1953) in South America, also explored countertransference more independently.

The sensitivity to the object relations of the analyst and the specific object relations in the psychoanalytic setting developed strongly in the 1940s. The Klein group was also stimulated by the description of projective identification (Klein, 1946). Projective identification became a development that strongly supported the theorising of countertransference, although Klein herself was initially suspicious and always very cautious (see Chapter 6). This reconsideration of countertransference then became a dominant trend, and even a developing orthodoxy, although with different emphases between the Kleinian and other groups.

In short, the concept suddenly became widened beyond merely the neurotic aspects of the analyst (Winnicott, 1949; Heimann, 1950; Little, 1951; Reich, 1951; Gitelson, 1952; Milner, 1952; Racker, 1953), and increasingly became a technical issue. Countertransference began to refer to the whole of the analyst's affective responses (Heimann, 1950; King, 1978); and a consensus developed amongst the strands of object-relations theory (Milner, 1952; Winnicott, 1955; Little, 1951; Balint,

1950).

With the rapid change after Freud's death in 1939, the suspicion in which countertransference was held began to abate, especially in this object-relations context. So by 1950, Paula Heimann could write in her key reappraisal:

> My thesis is that the analyst's emotional response to his patient within the analytic situation represents one of the most important tools for his work. The analyst's counter-transference is an instrument of research into the patient's unconscious (Heimann, 1950, p. 81).

Heimann used the term 'countertransference' to include *all* the feelings the analyst has towards her patient, because, '… the counter-transference is functioning as a delicate receiving apparatus (Money-Kyrle, 1956, p. 361). Roger Money-Kyrle was clearly making a distant allusion, as did Heimann, to Freud's (1912) likening of the analyst's unconscious as a 'receptive organ' to the patient's unconscious (quoted above, Chapter 1). This hint in Freud's 'recommendations' implied that unlike the surgeon, the analyst is in close emotional contact with the patient. If the analyst can be aware of his reactions to the patient, including the patient's transference, then he has access to the subjectivity in the patient.

Whilst Heimann made no reference to Klein in her 1950 paper, she did instead turn to Freud and his 'evenly suspended attention' (Freud, 1912) for support:

> We know that the analyst needs an evenly hovering attention in order to follow the patient's free associations, and that this enables him to listen simultaneously on many levels. He has to perceive the manifest and the latent meaning of his patient's words, the allusions and implications, the hints to former sessions, the references to childhood situations behind the description of current relationships, etc. By listening in this manner the analyst avoids the danger of becoming preoccupied with any one theme and remains receptive for the significance of changes in themes and of the sequences and gaps in the patient's associations (Heimann 1950, p, 82).

This paradigm shift usually associated with Heimann (1950) makes reference to Freud's notion of the analyst as an unconscious receiving apparatus:

> In my view Freud's demand that the analyst must 'recognize and master' his counter-transference does not lead to the conclusion that the counter-transference is a disturbing factor and that the analyst should become unfeeling and detached, but that he must use his emotional response as a key to the patient's unconscious (Heimann, 1950, p. 83).

She also claimed further support, 'The fact that the problem of the counter-transference has been put forward for discussion practically simultaneously by different workers indicates that the time is ripe for a more thorough research into the nature and function of the counter-transference' (p. 81n). Heimann referred to Ferenczi, and also to Alice Balint's paper in the *Internazionale Zeitschrift*, in 1936 which drew on Ferenczi. There had been a continuous, though underground, respect for these unconscious countertransference influences.

Winnicott, with his debt to Klein and his deep interest in the precise details of the analytic relationship, was a contributor with his paradox of an object experienced as both 'me' and 'not-me', a kind of merged state. He went as far as to reiterate Freud's 'there is no such thing as a baby' (Winnicott, 1960, p. 586n). This was captured by Margaret Little (1951), to understand the interactive aspects of 'transitional space', the in-between of the interpersonal in a two-person psychology:

> [T]ransference and counter-transference are not only syntheses by the patient and analyst acting separately, but, like the analytic work as a whole, are the result of a joint effort. We often hear of the mirror which the analyst holds up to the patient, but the patient holds one up to the analyst too. (Little, 1951, p. 37)

Thus the countertransference is a human encounter, but a specific one in which the analyst's mind is deeply affected by the patient's experiences that the analyst *feels*. It is more than playing a role; it is having a specific experience in the role. This conceptualisation was possible once the mechanism of projective identification had been described (Klein, 1946).

The paradigm shift had drawn upon the European tradition as brought to London in various moments, and had accumulated from various contacts, including the many émigrés.

The eventual shift in the *clinical use* of countertransference was articulated in several ways, not all consistent. For instance, in the US there has only more recently been a parallel shift. In contrast to Europe, the US had a very different psychoanalytic history. The Viennese diaspora spread out across the States to form a blanket hegemony of the classical ego-psychology school. This had set out to supplant (Kirsner, 1999) the indigenous and pluralist tradition already there. However, a paradigm shift has occurred in the US too, for different, though parallel, reasons from the 1970s onwards (Searles, 1979), looking back in part to Sullivan (Conci, 2010) in the 1930s and 1940s, before the ego-psychology 'invasion'. Recent interaction between the British and the US models of countertransference with their different histories has spawned a wide current debate, which we will partially cover later.

CHAPTER 5

Unconscious-to-unconscious How do they communicate?

As we saw (Chapter 1), Freud had early on puzzled over the eruption of passionate feelings in the analyst as discovered by Jung and Ferenczi. He described the importance of the analyst's unconscious being attuned to that of the patient's (Freud, 1912), but had little purchase on how such communication came about. Now, in the earliest stages of the new paradigm in the late 1940s, it was possible to exploit other developments in British psychoanalysis. These were contested in Britain and rejected elsewhere at this time, but now form an explanatory theory for understanding the creation of countertransference in the analyst. These theories come from the investigation and use of the so-called 'primitive mechanisms', splitting, projection and introjection, and projective identification, together with their effect on the coherence of the ego (or, in other words, the sense of the self's identity).

Cycles of projection and introjection

Heimann had contributed a significant paper in 1943 to the Controversial Discussions, delivered from the Kleinian camp. It was titled 'Some aspects of the role of introjection and projection in early development' (published a decade later as 'Certain functions of introjection and projection in early infancy'. Heimann had originally trained in Berlin around 1930, and came to Britain in 1934, when she then became an analysand of Klein's, and a loyal supporter. The part she played in the crucial Controversial Discussions (King and Steiner, 1991) was most prominent and effective.

In the published version of her paper on introjection and projection (written in 1943), she captured the interactions between minds in terms of this intimate and intruding way:

> Life is maintained through an organism's intake of foreign but useful matter and discharge of its own, but harmful, matter. Intake and discharge are most fundamental processes of any living organism. The mind, also a part of a living organism, is no exception to this rule: it achieves its adaptation and progress by employing throughout its existence the fundamental processes of introjection and projection (Heimann, 1952, p. 129).

This is almost a gastro-intestinal model of a relationship. However, this is a significant revision in 1952, and she says, with the benefit of Klein's 1946 introduction of splitting and projection of parts of the self (projective identification):

> It is not only in expelling an unsuitable external stimulus, which it proved a mistake, as it were, to take in, that the ego uses projection. When it discharges inner tensions, it projects something of its own. Thus projection relates to what was originally part of the self as well as to what was originally part of the outer world (Heimann, 1952, p. 125).

At this point, Heimann was still using the idea that the ego can split off parts of itself and project them with bad objects, etc. Nevertheless, by 1950, when Heimann wrote about countertransference, she had been becoming hesitant about Klein's theories. So, in 1950, Heimann could not easily take advantage of these theoretical developments, arising from the recent descriptions of the primitive, schizoid mechanisms, as recently described by Melanie Klein (1946).

Eventually, she disagreed deeply with Klein, and progressively more intensely, apparently over innate aggression, though there may have been more personal tensions (Grosskurth, 1986), which could connect with countertransference feelings in their own complex relationship; Heimann's analysis with Klein had been mingled with their professional relations as colleagues.

By 1955, Heimann had formally broken from the Klein group (Tonnesmann, 1989). So ironically, she was not easily able to use the theoretical basis – the primitive mechanisms of splitting, projection, introjection, and particularly projective identification – which were most obviously applicable to countertransference. It was then left to others to exploit the roles of projection and introjection in establishing a countertransference in a psychoanalysis. One notable contribution was Money-Kyrle's (1956). He pointedly referred in the title to his paper, to *normal* countertransference, and distinguished it from the deviations, about which he wrote that:

> [Unfortunately, the analyst] is not omniscient. In particular, his understanding fails whenever the patient corresponds too closely with some aspect of himself which he has not yet learnt to understand ... [W]hen that interplay between introjection and projection, which characterizes the analytic process, breaks down, the analyst may tend to get stuck in one or other of these two positions (1956, pp. 361-2).

His reference to two positions here is to the place of projection and introjection, similar to Heimann's emphasis. These mechanisms were to provide a means of communication at a very early level, before in fact any language had developed. In fact, a baby cries in its first days, and mother reacts with feelings of concern, worry, even panic, and all sorts of more mature responses. Baby has thus projected *something*, and mother has introjected it. This 'something' is not a physical thing, but a mental something.

Money-Kyrle, without making reference to the mother-baby instance, applied this early developmental model to the analytic situation:

> [T]here is a fairly rapid oscillation between introjection and projection. As the patient speaks, the analyst will, as it were, become introjectively identified with him, and having understood him inside, will reproject him and interpret (Money-Kyrle, 1956, p. 361).

He is in fact reiterating a model that might have come from Heimann at her most Kleinian. However, he added something; he added the idea of getting 'stuck' – stuck with an introjection that cannot be dropped, or stuck with a projection into the patient that cannot be recovered.

In the introjective stuck position, ill-understood aspects of the patient remain inside the analyst and continue to burden him after the session. Then, alternatively in the projective stuck position, aspects of the patient's experience, together with uncomprehended aspects of the analyst, will be projected back into the patient. When stuck in the projective position (with something of himself in the patient), he will experience a sense of depletion, 'often experienced as the loss of intellectual potency' (Money-Kyrle, 1956, p. 362), and he may become confused and feel stupid.

Feeling useless: an example

Money-Kyrle (1956, pp. 362-363) gave a clinical example of this process;

> [A male patient arrived very anxious because] he had not been able to work in his office. He had also felt vague on the way as if he might get lost or run over; and he despised himself for being useless (p. 362).

He presented quite consciously the experience of feeling useless. At first he used words, and the analyst made a link:

> Remembering a similar occasion, on which he had felt depersonalized over a week-end and dreamed that he had left his 'radar' set in a shop and would be unable to get it before Monday, I thought he had, in phantasy, left parts of his 'good self' in me. But I was not very sure of this, or of other interpretations I began to give (p. 362).

The analyst himself began to feel unsure now – about his interpretations. Perhaps he is making premature interpretations with a rather intellectual link – not a lively one. Perhaps he wanted to reassure himself, and so not have to feel the patient's uselessness:

> [The patient] soon began to reject them [the interpretations] all with a mounting degree of anger; and, at the same time, abused me for not helping. By the end of the session he was no longer depersonalized, but very angry and contemptuous instead. It was I who felt useless and bemused (Money-Kyrle, 1956, p. 362-363).

Perhaps it is understandable that the patient rejected the interpretation if the analyst did. But there is more than that. The patient became abusive about the lack of help, and used this method to arouse the *analyst's* feelings of uselessness:

> [The analyst] could not at once recognize it as corresponding with anything already understood in myself; and, for this reason, I was slow to get it out of me in the process of explaining, and so relieving it in him (Money-Kyrle, 1956, p. 363).

Here there is the typical interactive process between two minds. First, the patient felt useless. Then, by the end of the session, it had changed; the analyst felt useless, and the patient did not. This described the process of projective identification in which the patient, with a painful feeling of uselessness, projected that experience into the analyst. The analyst became disturbed and, feeling useless, lost his ability to understand what happened. In this instance, the analyst became 'stuck' in the introjective phase. He was left with his experience after the session, but later realised that though he was being useless that day, the patient was exploiting it and thus relieving himself. That situation was confirmed, and did improve:

> [The patient] was in the same mood at the beginning of the next [session] – still very angry and contemptuous. I then told him I thought he felt he had reduced me to the state of useless vagueness he himself had been in; and that he felt he had done this by having me 'on the mat', asking questions and rejecting the answers, in the way his legal father did. His response was striking. For the first time in two days, he became quiet and thoughtful. He then said this explained why he had been so angry with me yesterday: he had felt that all my interpretations referred to my illness and not to his (Money-Kyrle, 1956, p. 363).

The patient's state of mind changed as a direct result of the interpretation, so it seemed to strike something in the patient. It looks as though the patient could work out something about his own feelings and where they were. He had been struck by something arresting that the analyst said. It was an alive moment, and he had acquired a small bit of understanding, which represented an addition to his ego functioning.

This also illustrates an important technical point. There is a difference between helping the patient to feel better – which he undoubtedly did when he could change from feeling useless to feeling angry and contemptuous – and on the other hand, learning something – the specific method he used to make himself feel better.

However:

> [B]efore my patient's part in bringing it about could be interpreted, I had to do a silent piece of self-analysis involving the discrimination of two things which can be felt as very similar: my own sense of incompetence at having lost the thread, and my patient's contempt for his impotent self, which he felt to be in me (p. 363).

So, the analyst's work is to analyse himself, not just the patient, in order to determine what feelings belong to the patient, and what feelings belong to the analyst that the patient could make some use of defensively. This 'double' work of the analyst could then help clarify for the patient how the uselessness *in the analyst*, was a part of his own experience, as well. The patient could then, in turn, make his own discrimination between his experience as he felt it, and his experience seen as the analyst's experience.

Now, a secondary experience the patient had at this moment was that although he could not himself tolerate feeling useless, his analyst could tolerate it (if slowly); this contributed no doubt to the patient's increased tolerance of his own feeling of being useless. The patient's ability to work through this projection was thus directly dependent on the analyst separating two things that felt very similar:

- the analyst's own sense of incompetence having lost the thread, and

- the patient's contempt for *his* impotent self, which he now felt to be in the analyst.

This is one of the really difficult situations – when a patient's projection meets something vulnerable in the analyst[4].

The analyst here was required by the patient to contain the patient's feelings of uselessness. Because of certain aspects of the analyst's own personality, it seems the analyst could himself feel useless. However, because something in the analyst matched something in the patient, the analyst became

---

4   This meeting of unconscious personality difficulties has subsequently been highlighted by, for instance, Bernard Brandschaft et al. (2010), as 'pathological accommodation'. Such unconscious 'meeting' (or accommodation) is a key pillar in the understanding of psychoanalytic interrsubjectivity by the recent Relational school of psychoanalysis.

confused, lost temporarily his insight into himself and the patient, and failed to understand fully what was going on. He did not identify the feelings at first, but that was the step that Money-Kyrle says was necessary.

This is a clear enough statement of a view of countertransference based on the concepts of projection, introjection and identification, and how it may be used in practice at this time. The use of countertransference may involve learning about oneself, 'by discovering new patterns in a patient, the analyst can make "post-graduate" progress in his own analysis' (Money-Kyrle, 1956, p. 365, note 4). In another interesting note, Money-Kyrle confided:

> How exactly a patient does succeed in imposing a phantasy and its corresponding affect upon his analyst in order to deny it in himself is a most interesting problem. I do not think we need assume some form of extrasensory communication; but the communication can be of a pre-verbal and archaic kind similar perhaps to that used by gregarious animals in which the posture or call of a single member will arouse a corresponding affect in the rest. In the analytic situation, a peculiarity of communications of this kind is that, at first sight, they do not seem as if they had been made by the patient at all. The analyst experiences the affect as being

his own response to something. The effort involved is in differentiating the patient's contribution from his own (Money-Kyrle, 1956, p. 366, note 10).

The 'democratic' context

To a considerable extent, the period in which the revision of countertransference took place was the period of the Cold War when the idea of 'democracy' was highlighted for cultural and political advantage. This background helped the revision in views on countertransference, and the revision of authority in both society at large and in the psychoanalytic setting. This inevitably led to egalitarian views of many therapeutic forms, including psychoanalysis, and an intention to give a stronger place to the patient's voice. In addition, the emergence of an understanding of projective identification led to a sense of greater familiarity with the unconscious-to-unconscious communication that had puzzled Freud.

But even Alice Balint's (1936) paper had sought to privilege a respect for the patient by suggesting that such honesty – expressing one's own feelings – on the part of the analyst is helpful and in keeping with the respect for truth inherent in psycho-analysis. It emphasises an attitude of fairness. Other analysts too have claimed that it makes the analyst more 'human' when he expresses his feelings to his patient and that it helps him to build up a 'human' relationship with him. Ferenczi's experiments assumed that knowledge would operate two-way. Balint (1936) stressed that both the patient and the analyst have libidinal investments in each other and in the analysis. Little (1951) examined this question too, and recommended that the analyst occasionally share her analysis of her own feelings with the patient.

In classical psychoanalysis, only the patient is known, and that was in line with the requirement for a blank-screen analyst. So, in the interests of equality, and perhaps a full intimacy, Ferenczi revised that; perhaps the setting should be arranged such that it could be reversed. Whereas, normally, the analyst is in a position to know the patient, reversing the physical position of analyst and patient would reverse who gets to know whom. In fact, Alice Balint (1936) reviewed Ferenczi's experiments, recommending, ultimately, that the classical technique should be adhered to in most cases, but not all. This tradition, coming from Ferenczi's clinical experimentation (1988) and continued by Balint in London (Balint & Balint, 1939; Balint, 1950), has been represented by the British Independent group of analysts (Kohon, 1986; Rayner, 1991; Stewart, 1996).

However, Michael Balint also suggested that the understanding of the patient's transference and of the analyst's countertransference do not exhaust the necessary work:

[Descriptions of the states of the two individuals]

> remain incomplete through the neglect of an essential
> feature, namely, that all these phenomena happen in an
> inter-relation between two individuals, in a constantly
> changing and developing object-relation (1950, p. 123).

Balint's tradition is a premonitory hint of the later development
of the idea of the analytic field (Baranger and Baranger,
1983; Ferro, 1999); and of Ogden's idea of the 'analytic third'
(Ogden, 1999) though Ogden acknowledges more of a debt
to Winnicott than Balint, (Chapter 7, where this approach will
be called co-constructivist). Balint's idea of the harmonious
inter-relation was conceived at the beginning of the current
'democratic era', as it began to form in reaction to National
Socialism and to Stalinism. Interestingly, these later views on
the countertransference, as a field of mutual influence, took
root more in the US.

The intra-psychic approach

In contrast to the Ferenczi-Balint tradition, I return here to
the projection-introjection approach to understanding the
communication between the two unconscious minds. Edna
O'Shaughnessy presents one claim:

> It is now widely held that, instead of being about the
> patient's intrapsychic dynamics, interpretations should
> be about the interaction of patient and analyst at an
> intrapsychic level (O'Shaughnessy, 1983, p. 281).

This can be called the intra-psychic approach. The *inner* world constitutes a subject, it is not the inter-relationship that does so. Rather, the two inner subjective worlds constitute the interaction.

The intra-psychic approach keeps the subjectivities separate, even though at times those entities may become less separate as they influence and encroach on each other. For each subjectivity, the sense of being an out-there presence for the other is a core ingredient of identity – perhaps *the* core ingredient of an identity. The two minds interact in the immediate present, emphasising the here-and-now process; as Ezriel put it succinctly in 1956: 'only such forces as exist at a certain time can have effects at that time' (Ezriel, 1956. p. 35). Psychoanalysis is ahistorical, like natural science. In fact, the focus on the 'immediacy' of interpretation started early. That focus may also have been one of the influences that underlay these British developments. That is to say, an emphasis on the play of forces in the immediately present process throws attention towards both the transference and the countertransference. Strachey's classic paper on interpretation in 1934 said:

> [I]nterpretations must always be directed to the 'point of urgency'. At any given moment some particular id-impulse will be in activity; this is the impulse that is

susceptible of mutative interpretation at that time, and no other one (Strachey, 1934, p. 150).

Strachey conveyed what happens 'at that time':

> The analytic situation is all the time threatening to degenerate into a 'real' situation. But this actually means the opposite of what it appears to. It means that the patient is all the time on the brink of turning the real external object (the analyst) into the archaic one; that is to say, he is on the brink of projecting his primitive introjected imagos on to him. In so far as the patient actually does this, the analyst becomes like anyone else that he meets in real life – a phantasy object (Strachey, 1934, p. 146).

Transference emerges from *constantly active* unconscious phantasy in the analysand, which interacts with constantly active unconscious phantasy in the psychoanalyst. The latter may in reality begin to take up such a role, such as behaving with a harsh super-ego-like father, perhaps.

Edward Glover complained about this, and resisted this British development (leaving the British Society altogether in 1944). He severely castigated the 'Klein system' as he called it:

> [B]y their [revised] theories of the "uninterrupted influence" of the concepts of fixation and regression,

they have abandoned the Freudian theory of
neurosogenesis (Glover, 1945, p. 118).

The Kleinian view is that unconscious phantasies of primitive,
archaic objects (Isaacs, 1952 [1943]) remain constantly active
in the 'deeper layers' of the unconscious. Glover disagreed,
supporting the classical view that phantasies of archaic objects
arise from regression (and fixation) *at times of stress*. Glover's
view, aligned with the Viennese position at the time, would
deny that there are equivalent primitive phantasies in the
analyst waiting to be activated by the patient's unconscious
projections.

Mutual confidences. Despite Ferenczi's experiments, the origins of
the new views on countertransference have led many object-
relations analysts to debate and refute the suggestion that
analysts might share their feelings with their patients (also see
Casement, 1985; Bollas, 1989). Nevertheless, the recognition
that the analyst's style and the atmosphere engendered become
a playful creativity between patient and analyst has developed
strong roots in the work of some of the British Independent
School. It appears to offer the patient an equal partnership
in a process that restores a normal mutuality in the 'affective
response' of one to the other. When this mutuality seems to be
interrupted, the analyst will, modestly, tend to assume that the
patient feels the analyst has missed something, and will then
engage in an internal supervision (Casement, 1985).

Contrast with classical analysis. The classical approach of remaining sceptical and suspicious of the countertransference at this time relied upon Hartmann's (1939) idea of the 'autonomous ego', an area of ego function that is spared the conflicts over the instincts. Conflicts then arise only intermittently when primitive conflicts erupt. It has been clear for a long time (Zetzel, 1956) that this approach remained impervious to the position on unconscious phantasy argued by Susan Issacs for the Kleinians:

> It would appear implicit in [Hartmann's] argument that conflict-free or autonomous ego functions are relatively, if not absolutely, independent of unconscious significance. Susan Isaacs (1952), on the other hand, states, "In our view reality thinking cannot operate without concurrent and supporting unconscious fantasies. The fact that fantasy thinking and reality thinking have a distinct character when fully developed does not necessarily imply that reality operates quite independently of unconscious fantasy." This would imply that for Melanie Klein and her followers no mental activity, however functionally free, can be devoid of unconscious significance (Zetzel, 1956, p. 114).

There is an absolute difference of opinion on whether a

person can be regarded as ever operating outside the zone of unconscious phantasies and conflicts, and in a conflict-free autonomous way that is spared the interference of the unconscious. Hartman and ego-psychologists at the time had decided that normal activity does operate outside the conflicted neurotic zone of unconscious phantasies; Kleinians, so influential at the time in British psychoanalysis, decided that nothing is outside that conflicted zone. Those influenced by Kleinians, including Strachey (1934) and Ezriel (1956), accepted the constant unconscious influence, and so developed the intra-psychic approach. The ego-psychologists, on the other hand, claimed the ego in health potentially operates independently from the unconscious conflicts. Therefore, they argued that under normal conditions countertransference does not interfere and can be removed from consideration.

This yawning gap from the 1950s onwards determined a wide difference of opinion on countertransference. The classical psychoanalyst was expected to operate within the autonomous, conflict-free zone – that is to say, he is free of countertransference influences from his unconscious. The patient, likewise, must be helped to occupy his own autonomous zone as much as possible. Indeed, the activity of analysis during the sessions is expected to maintain an autonomy from the unconscious influence, by the formation of what was called a 'treatment alliance' between analyst and analysand. Hence, countertransference has no place, because if it intrudes, it interrupts the proper working of their un-conflicted alliance.

Implicitly, transference in this classical view comes from the past, through fixation points and regression to them; and so countertransference emerges when the analyst's incompletely analysed fixation points complement those points in the patient. On the other hand, in the intra-psychic view, transference is from the unconscious to the present, rather than from the past to the present. So, countertransference then matches transference, being the mobilisation of a response that complements the patient's transference[5] and expresses unconscious meanings with the conscious ones.

The unconscious as a receptive organ

It should be clear how those tracing unconscious phantasy to the present unconscious find it more consistent to recognise the impact on the analyst. In that way, Heimann could see how this immediate here-and-now process of transference and countertransference reveals the core phantasies that impel the

---

5   Racker (1968), in the first generation of revisionists, described concordant and complementary countertransferences. These varieties correlate with a British pro-jection-introjection model, such that 'concordant' means the patient has projected a part of himself, and the analyst feels, speaks and behaves as if he were that part of the patient (for instance, the analyst feels the anxiety instead of the patient), whereas the 'complementary' form implies the patient has projected an internal object that is significant at the moment, and the analyst plays a part in relation to the patient's ego that recreates the internal relationship in the external setting (for instance, the analyst comes to play the part of the patient's super-ego).

personality of the patient. It can therefore serve as a source of information for the psychoanalyst to understand the core phantasies that represent wishes, conflicts and defences at the moment of the analysis.

Money-Kyrle (1956) called the analyst's unconscious a delicate receiving apparatus, clearly following Freud:

> If the analyst is in fact disturbed, it is also likely that the patient has unconsciously contributed to this result, and is in turn disturbed by it. So we have three factors to consider: first, the analyst's emotional disturbance, for he may have to deal with this silently in himself before he can disengage himself sufficiently to understand the other two; then the patient's part in bringing it about; and finally its effect on him. Of course, all three factors may be sorted out in a matter of seconds, and then indeed the counter-transference is functioning as a delicate receiving apparatus (Money-Kyrle, 1956, p. 361).

The receiving apparatus may need constant tuning, through self-analysis. The analyst is obliged, paradoxically, to be aware of what he is not aware, and in fact dependent on the patient giving indications, unconscious indications, of what is going on. In the case of Money-Kyrle's example of uselessness, earlier in this chapter, the patient had conveyed his own confusion when criticised by his father – indeed this was conveyed in verbal statements, but also in the process of emotional interaction between the two players. Because it was powerfully projected and enacted, it was not easy to grasp the significance quickly. In fact, Money-Kyrle's piece of self-analysis took place after the session, and in this instance could only take place when the analyst was freed from the unconscious pressure from the patient.

Moreover, this is a continuous process. Each intrapsychic system is a system in its own right; neither is closed, and each depends to some extent on the other. As Susan Issacs expressed it more than 70 years ago:

> [O]ur material changes from moment to moment. Our patient's thoughts and feelings and intentions do not stay still while we examine and compare them. The changes occurring are themselves part of our evidence. They not only bring us new data, but are themselves data by which we gain understanding of the patient's history and present life (Isaacs, 1939, p. 156).

In view of the constant interchange of projections and introjections, each intrapsychic world is highly influenced in the moment, and sometimes in the long-term (we hope at least one of them will be influenced in the long-term). Heimann's descriptions suggest we think about each mind as a system that operates processes of incorporation and evacuation.

Bion (1962b) adopted Heimann's metaphor of the mind as a digestive system, a psychic swallowing, digesting, and eliminating. Paula Heimann was one of Bion's training supervisors. Bion, however, developed the model beyond Heimann and Money-Kyrle to describe the concept of containing. A particular feature of this kind of model of intersubjectivity is that an element of one subjectivity goes *inside* the other, as Money-Kyrle described, but then comes out again in a modified form. Bion described this in order to link this particularly intimate kind of conjoining to Oedipal phantasies and conflicts. Bion said, also mimicking Freud:

> The mother's capacity for reverie is the receptor organ for the infant's harvest of self-sensation gained by its conscious (Bion, 1962a, p. 309).

But not only mothers, the analyst must do the same and cultivate the state of reverie. Bion thought that the analyst has to use his own reverie as that receptor organ/receiving apparatus. This is not merely a phenomenon of disturbed patients. Brenman Pick gave the following example:

> Consider a patient bringing particularly good or particularly bad news; say, the birth of a new baby or a death in the family. Whilst such an event may raise

complex issues requiring careful analysis, in the first instance the patient may not want an interpretation, but a response; the sharing of pleasure or of grief. And this may be what the analyst intuitively wishes for too. Unless we can properly acknowledge this in our interpretation, interpretation itself either becomes a frozen rejection, or is abandoned and we feel compelled to act non-interpretively and be 'human' (Brenman Pick, 1985, p. 160).

This is an interaction between two 'open' systems.

These explorations of the interaction of two subjectivities, the intra-psychic approach, contrast with the two other trends. First is classical ego-psychology, where the encroachment of countertransference is a sign of pathology to be suppressed. Second is the position forecast by the Balints' understanding of the joint creation of an interactive domain, i.e. the co-constructivists, as I shall call them in a chapter soon to come (Chapter 7).

CHAPTER 6

Debate – Klein/Heimann
What unacknowledged agreement
did they reach?

Curiously, although the impetus for the revision in views of countertransference was given a spur by Melanie Klein's influential concept of projective identification, Klein herself remained cautious and sceptical of countertransference. Heimann had been, up to the time she wrote her paper in 1950, a protégé of Melanie Klein's, and she had provided enthusiastic and effective support to Klein during the Controversial Discussions of the 1940s (King and Steiner, 1991). In January 1935, Paula Heimann had started her analysis with Melanie Klein. Though trained as a psychoanalyst in Berlin, she read a paper for her membership of the British Psychoanalytical Society in 1939, on a patient with delusional experiences about being occupied by demons. The paper was given, in part, in order to state a Kleinian position on internal objects. It was also a response to a paper given by Anna Freud on sublimation, the first paper Anna Freud gave to the scientific meetings of the British Psychoanalytical Society (see Hinshelwood, 1997b).

In 1949, Heimann wrote her paper on countertransference for the IPA Congress in Zurich, though Klein apparently advised her not to. Heimann did not take that advice and presented the paper to the Congress, publishing it in 1950. The paper contained no reference to Klein at all, and their difference was not made public in the 1950 paper. There ensued a period when Klein and Heimann moved apart. Klein may also have felt it best not to make her criticisms of Heimann public either. For whatever reason, Klein therefore disagreed with Heimann's radical paper, aggravating a tension between them, from which their professional solidarity never recovered (Grosskurth, 1986).

Spillius put Klein's position like this, 'Klein thought that such extension [of the use of countertransference] would open the door to claims by analysts that their own deficiencies were caused by their patients' (Spillius, 1992, p. 61). The irony is therefore that Klein, who had done so much to support and develop the object-relations point of view in British psychoanalysis, remained reluctant to accept the revision of countertransference towards a more object-relations view. Late in her life, in 1958, Klein said in discussion with a group of young colleagues:

> You know, of course that the patient is bound to stir certain feelings in the analyst and that this varies

> according to the patient's attitude... though there
> are of course feelings at work in the analyst which
> he has to become aware of. I have never found that
> countertransference has helped me to understand my
> patient better. If I may put it like this, I have found that
> it helped me to understand myself better (Klein, 1958,
> unpublished, quoted in Spillius 2007, p. 78).

Ambivalently, she acknowledged that the analyst's feelings do vary according to the patient's attitude; but at the same time, she denied that much understanding of the patient comes from it.

Klein did not take it the step further that Money-Kyrle (1956) did when he said the analyst must 'do a small piece of self-analysis', and apply that new bit of self-knowledge to the way the patient had activated it. Though he admitted this might often have to be after the session, Klein simply believed that countertransference led to mistakes:

> I mean it has so much to do with the analyst that I
> really feel that my own experience... is rather to find
> out within myself when I made a mistake (Klein, 1958,
> unpublished, quoted in Spillius 2007, p.78).

This was again from her discussion with young analysts in 1958. It is not entirely off target, but it depends what follows from making a mistake. Did she dismiss the mistake as *nothing* to do with the context that the analyst is in (she is with a patient), so that countertransference is entirely a personal matter?

She did know that the analyst's reactions were potentially signposts for the analysis, because she left notes indicating that possibility. In her Archive in the Wellcome Library in London, she gives the text of comments she made in a discussion at an IPA Congress in London in 1953. In response to a paper given by Wilfred Bion on schizophrenia (see Hinshelwood, 2008), she described:

> [T]he patient's violent processes of splitting the analyst and pushing into him parts of his self and of his impulses – a process which I have named projective identification – has a most strenuous effect on the analyst.

> Dr. Bion has illustrated the way in which his patient split him by the instance of the two opposite buttons which the patient wanted to press in the lift. Such processes are apt to make the analyst tired, sleepy, and stir up strong resistance against the work in him. The point I wish to emphasise is that only by studying the processes of projective identification in their roots in the first few months of life, as well as their implications, that the analyst can cope in himself with

this particular counter-transference difficulty (quoted in Hinshelwood, 2008, p. 109).

It would seem that Klein is in fact pointing to the need to study the processes affecting the analyst (i.e. projective identification as it created countertransference), and especially so with schizophrenic patients. In other words, the analyst's state of tension is a pointer to the negativity in the patient, and *not only* a mistake by the analyst.

A question arises then about Klein's reticence in writing about countertransference, especially as the study of countertransference helped, during her lifetime, to an understanding of the importance of her concept of projective identification. Why did she not publish more of the views she had expressed in these papers, left only to be archived? It was not that she decided they were wrong, since she did mention them briefly again in 1959:

> Even the patient's co-operation, which allows for an analysis of very deep layers of the mind, of destructive impulses, and of persecutory anxiety, may up to a point be influenced by the urge to satisfy the analyst and to be loved by him. The analyst who is aware of this will analyse the infantile roots of such wishes; otherwise, in identification with his patient, the early need for reassurance may strongly influence his

counter-transference and therefore his technique. This identification may also easily tempt the analyst to take the mother's place and give in to the urge immediately to alleviate his child's (the patient's) anxieties (Klein, 1959, p. 225-226).

She is aware of the impact on the analyst of the patient's deep need to please. She indicates that it only leads to a mistake in technique, and she is a hairs-breadth from acknowledging the indicative function of the countertransference. When Klein wrote the archived 'Notes on countertransference' (quoted above) in 1953, there had been a considerable history to her relationship with Heimann, and Klein was greatly indebted to Heimann's fierce defence of Kleinian ideas in the Controversial Discussions (King and Steiner, 1991).

Despite her reluctance, Klein's followers have taken a major part in forging the new view of countertransference, and emphasising the relational aspects of the transference–countertransference (Bion, 1959; Segal, 1975; Rosenfeld, 1987). Moreover, they have heavily used one of Klein's most central concepts, projective identification, as fundamental to this emotional responsiveness.

Clinical rigour: Heimann's warning

Despite Klein's disagreement – or possibly because of it – Heimann eventually admitted some reservations about how her recommendations had been taken up. The growing enthusiasm for the kind of access afforded by countertransference to the patient's unconscious transference led her to a concern at a possible over-confidence in the use of one's feelings.

Heimann's warning. So, 10 years later, Heimann returned to the debate, and there is an echo of Klein's concern, that the use of countertransference can merely attribute the analyst's defensiveness to the patient. She wrote:

> I may mention that I have had occasion to see that my [earlier] paper also caused some misunderstanding in that some candidates, who referring to my paper for justification, uncritically, based their interpretations on their feelings. They said in reply to any query 'my countertransference', and seemed disinclined to check their interpretations against the actual data in the analytic situation (Heimann, 1960, p. 153).

Here she positively chastised analysts for not checking 'their interpretations against the actual data of the analytic situation'. It appeared to her that analysts, especially inexperienced ones, can abuse the use of countertransference. The wild and uncritical use of the analyst's feelings needs to be tempered. This appeal for caution, and a checking process on the use of countertransference, was published by Heimann in the year that Klein died[6]. We can only wonder if Klein approved of Heimann's second (1960) paper, its warning, its recommendation, and the use to which it has subsequently been put, if in fact she read it before she died.

So, this later recommendation of Heimann's, in 1960, was that in order to use the countertransference reliably, we should check it against the actual data in the analytic situation. As Bion had already remarked in conformity with Heimann's later requirement, 'Evidence for interpretations has to be found in the countertransference and in the actions and free associations of the patients' (Bion, 1954, p. 113).

Constant enactment

Using that checking device means a piece of material can be looked at from two points of view *in the session*:

- the *content* of the immediate free associative material, and

- the transference interaction (or, *engagement*) of the moment.

In practice, each is checked against the other. The best clinical work analysts do can then be assessed according to whether these two different perspectives are combined. It means there

---

6   Heimann's paper was published in March 1960, some six months before Klein's death in September.

is an intrinsic triangulation ready to hand in the clinical session (see also the research use of triangulation in Hinshelwood 2013a). So, in an on-going therapeutic process a psychoanalyst has a dual perspective – content and process. The *process* of the transference-countertransference engagement can replay the *content* of the associations in a little 'drama' for two actors in the session.

We have reached a point where the enactment of unconscious emotional dramas by *both* parties is inevitable, by virtue of the fact that both parties are emotionally responding people. As Joseph (1987, 1988), O'Shaughnessy (1992) and Carpy (1989) have suggested, we may have to recognize that a degree of enactment is almost inevitable; part of a continuing process that analysts can come to recognize (Feldman, 1997).

In the following brief example, the content in the form of a dream displays something that occurs in another form as well – in the drama played out in the process of presenting the dream:

> A colleague presented at a conference a dream from the middle of an analysis, most of which is not relevant here. The dream was simply: *A caravanserai in the middle of a desert.* The psychoanalyst found herself full of interesting ideas, but a bit perplexed because the patient had no associations or any affective response

to the dream even when asked. There was therefore an interactive process here between the two states of mind (analyst and analysand) both expressed in the telling of the dream – the analyst's intra-psychic state became more lively, and the analysand's less lively. The point is that the dream represented visually a 'desert' as well as the 'oasis' (i.e. the caravanserai). But that division – desert/oasis – was also represented in the psychic enactment – the two minds, one more lively and the other less so. Thus the content of the dream and the enactment between the psychoanalytic partners converged [my summary of the conference presentation– RDH].

This dual perspective of content and process is quintessentially a psychoanalytic occurrence. It requires listening not just to the verbal content, but also 'with the third ear' as we say, to pick up the intuited, 'felt' nuances of the presentation, as we exist (live) within the encounter with the patient. 'We analyse,' as Segal said, 'the dreamer not the dream' (quoted in Quinidoz, 2009, p. 94). Analysing the dreamer entails both the content of the dream and the process of the dreamer's presentation, which enacts the transference-countertransference engagement.

A long time ago, Glover expressed much the same view. It was rooted in the suspicion of countertransference that was dominant and accepted at the time:

> … to preoccupy oneself with the dream-material to the exclusion of a pressing transference re-enactment would merit a certain amount of self-inspection, on the grounds that the seemingly impersonal nature of dream-production may afford the analyst the same respite from unpleasantness as it does the patient (Glover, 1927, p. 505).

So Segal's comment echoed this concern about mechanical dream interpretation – or indeed any symbolic interpretation which is 'detrimental to the recognition of alive moments of emotional contact' (as Spillius put it). Segal described in considerable detail that the bringing of a dream may be more important than the content of the dream (Segal, 1981, 1991).

The act of bringing a dream may be an enactment in itself, an evacuation, a projective identification, a predictive commentary on the interaction in the session *after* the dream is dreamt, pleasing the analyst, and so on. It is extremely convenient (and shall we say, calming/deadening) for the psychoanalyst to then take up the content, whilst failing to learn from the joint enactment unfolding in the presentation. By doing so, he enters into a process with the patient that diverts the attention from the patient's need and towards enacting the evacuation of whatever motive. Segal's approach increasingly moved from the importance of the dream's content, to the *process* of bringing the dream. So, countertransference points a finger not just at the analyst's own mental functioning, but at the wider, and implied, importance of the interaction between the two partners to the encounter. One could say that to approach countertransference in a seemingly impersonal way can afford a similar respite from something unpleasant for the analyst as well as the patient.

Heimann's (1960) recommendation to use the content as a support to the use of countertransference process was restated by Busch, 'I worked with the transference throughout this material, and used my countertransference reactions as a backdrop to my interpretations' (Busch and Schmidt-Hellerau, 2004, p. 702). Whether the associations check the countertransference, or the countertransference checks the content of associations, the significant occurrence is when the two perspectives converge on one inferred narrative.

Gabbard (1996, pp. 262-263) reported a session with an unmarried woman who was alternately desiring of him and angry with him. The analyst had a strong reaction to her, but needed the evidence of the material (her dreams and phantasies) as well, to understand his reaction, and what they were enacting between them. After one occasion when she saw the previous (woman) patient leaving, she accused the psychoanalyst of deliberately causing her jealousy. Gabbard wrote:

> As I sat in session after session with her, engaging in my own process of reverie and self enquiry, I had a persistent feeling that she was dangerous, that she somehow wished to destroy me, and that I had to be on my guard with her.
>
> A dream she brought into the analysis just before a one-week absence of mine shed further light on what was transpiring between us. In the dream, Ms. D was standing in a shower washing male genitals that were unattached to a body. In her associations to the dream, Ms. D commented that she had read in the New York Times that they were arresting prostitutes in Manhattan and then printing the names of the men who visited them. She then told me, "I have a fantasy of taking you to the cleaners." She went on to say, "It must be related to literally castrating you. I can see you standing around missing your vital parts. But I don't want to leave here feeling I damaged you. I want to make sure everything's in its place. I don't want to be castrating toward you. I'm terribly afraid I'll damage you and lose you."

We can see here a correspondence between the analyst's countertransference, his sense of danger, and the patient's own fear of doing damage – an explicit dream about castrating a man. A little later, she was crying:

> "My father always said no man would put up with me. What I fear is that you'll see that behind my wish to seduce you and to become your lover is a desire to bring you down. I derive such a sense of power over men when I have sex with them. I feel like I literally bring them to their knees. I reduce them to my level."

There is a correspondence between

(a) the initial *countertransference* reaction of being in danger, and

(b) the *content*, the dream of being damaging by castration.

Thus a correspondence between two perspectives can be sensibly combined – 'The patient's dream and her associations had made it clearer to me why I felt a sense of danger and needed to be on my guard with her' (Gabbard, 1996, p. 263). The content and countertransference held a common inferred meaning.

Naturally, errors will occur, but the meaning is checked in this way by matching the two sources against each other.

CHAPTER 7

Co-constructed intersubjectivity
Where did ego-psychology go?

This chapter will consider the alternative development in the revision of countertransference. This emphasis on intersubjectivity was developed in the US (the co-constructivist approach), and had its origins in the gradually forming network of developments to come out of the declining dominance of ego-psychology. They are not yet clearly defined, but mapping those developments is not the purpose of this book.

In the US, the co-constructivist or intersubjectivist development began in the 1970s. However, the broad trends whose eventual divergence resulted in separate understandings of countertransference had been well underway in 1950. The intra-psychic model, arising earlier and within the object-relations schools of psychoanalysis, was not easily absorbed into the assumptions of psychoanalysis in the US. As a result, a new development, which we will call the co-constructivist model, has developed. It assumes an undifferentiated primary narcissism at birth, in contrast to the emphasis in Britain on very early established relations with objects. These two developments

create limitations, as well as opportunities, for a revised view
of the nature and origins of the countertransference.

The dominance of ego-psychology

The development of ego-psychology in Vienna was transported
to North America in the 1940s. There, a contest ensued between
the immigrant Viennese and the more indigenous American
interpersonal views. On the whole, the Viennese approach
supervened (Kirsner, 1999). Its characteristic, based on the
drive theory of the functioning of the ego and its defences, is
a progressive objectification of the subject. The mechanisms
of defence were no longer the spontaneous creativity of a
troubled living subject, but mechanical descriptions of forces
in conflict that were inherently instinctual and non-personal.
Reactive responses to the mechanical/technical approach of
psychoanalysis in North America post-WW2 were quite rapid,
and in part looked back to earlier traditions, such as William
Alison White and Harry Stack Sullivan. From the 1940s, the
hegemony of Viennese ego-psychology, with drive theory at
its core, delayed any reconsideration of countertransference
much longer than it did in Europe.

In addition, in the US, from the 1940s, the close affinity with
medicine led to a convergence between psychoanalytic and
medical approaches. Whilst the standard medical approach is
to fit patients to a diagnosis leading seamlessly to orthodox and

proven treatments, the same applied to psychoanalysis leads to the use of metapsychological theories as if they were medical diagnoses – persons are fitted to theories. Adolph Meyer (Lamb, 2014) was a psychiatrist who successfully influenced a psychodynamic approach within US psychiatry in the first half of the 20th century, when he sought to sensitize psychiatrists to patients' experience by promoting psychoanalysis within the psychiatric services. Both these processes, the medicalisation of psychoanalysis and the psychodynamic sensitisation of psychiatry, resulted in an extraordinary dominance for psychoanalysts within mental health provision in North America for a period of several decades.

The eventual problem with ego-psychology was its over-mechanistic approach to human experience, and the exclusion of the psychoanalyst's experience, behind his blank screen, from serious consideration (Fromm, 1970; Kohut, 1971). When contextual factors in North America led to the decline of ego-psychology from the 1980s onwards, countertransference did begin to be debated. That change was not initially because of new ideas. It was because new ideas and approaches had to be found to re-orient the classical ideas of ego-psychology. The newer developments may also have been supported by a combination of rhetoric about democracy in the wider culture, together with the social constructionism of post-modernism.

In search of new sources

Objectification on a medical pattern has latterly been disastrous for ego-psychology, and has led to many attempts to regenerate psychoanalysis in the United States along other lines, most of which seem to be coming together in terms of a respect for the intersubjectivity of the analyst-analysand relationship. In the last few decades, the development of a 'Relational' tradition has occurred in the US – associated with the names of Bernard Brandschaft, Stephen Mitchell, Jay Greenberg, and many others. Brandschaft (see Brandschaft et al., 2010) was an early prospector for new gold, once it appeared that ego-psychology and drive theory were waning. That trend looked in part to the object-relations tradition (Brandschaft was instrumental in inducing Wilfred Bion to emigrate to Los Angeles), and also to the work of the earlier American analysts, with the emphasis on the cultural environment (Harry Stack Sullivan, Erich Fromm, Frieda Fromm-Reichman). Self-psychology was one of the stations on the way, trying to get back to the experience of the patient in the room, an 'experience-near' stance.

The attempts initially have produced approaches of inter-subjectivism (Atwood and Stolorow, 1984, Ogden 1984, Renik 1993a) and relational psychoanalysis (Greenberg and Michell, 1983, Mitchell 1988). These new developments were in order to move away from the stereotyping procedure of the classical approach to psychoanalysis. It was more humane to recognise a psychoanalyst as having relations of a more personal kind with his patients. The espousal of countertransference has therefore been a part of the overall reaction against the excessive mechanisation of psychoanalysis.

These developments have only weakly adopted the crucial core of the British object-relations approach – that core being the central notion of displacing the primacy of impulse-satisfaction in favour of the object related to. Nevertheless, they have tended to adapt various later British analysts, notably Winnicott, Fairbairn and Bion, who have emphasised relations over drives and defences. Ferenczi, whose influence was quiescent during the Soviet period in Hungary, had emerged after 1990, and is now once again influential.

Some influence on the co-constructivist approach in the US was absorbed from British psychoanalysts. Balint (1950) had carried some of Ferenczi's ideas all through, having stressed the 'creating [of] a proper atmosphere for the patient by the analyst' (p. 123), and asserted that each analyst is unique and contributes his own atmosphere to the particular analysis. He comes close to the relational view, emphasising the 'interplay of transference and counter-transference' (p. 123), which forms something superordinate to the individuals. Balint's general approach to the patient in the context of the analytic encounter was also echoed in Winnicott's injunction 'to avoid breaking up this natural process by making interpretations' (Winnicott, 1969, p. 711). Winnicott increasingly saw the transference-countertransference as a delicate arena of its own which was evolved by both parties, as a version of transitional space. Making interpretations interrupts a natural process. 'I think I interpret mainly to let the patient know the limits of my understanding. The principle is that it is the patient and only the patient who has the answers' (p. 711).

There had always been a small group of classical Freudians in London, under Anna Freud's leadership, who were perforce in contact with and stimulated by those colleagues in Britain promoting an object-relations point of view. Perhaps it was easiest, therefore, for Anna Freud's group to render the new view of countertransference into a more classical language. For instance, Sandler later endorsed something like that more progressive view:

> [T]he psychoanalyst can be regarded as an instrument, a sort of probe into the psychoanalytic situation, that organizes the experience the analyst has in interaction with his patients through the formation of unconscious theoretical structures. The probe can be withdrawn from the situation and the theories which have been formed can be examined (Sandler, 1983, p. 38).

Sandler is here describing the analyst as activated to play a role, not just displayed on a 'screen' but actually playing the role. There is an inevitable role-responsiveness (Sandler and Sandler, 1987), implying an accommodating response, which, however, was given only token acceptance in the US context.

Crucial characteristics

A number of influences from within psychoanalysis and from without have contributed to the new developments in the co-constructivist approach.

Authenticity: The overarching direction is, increasingly, the authenticity of the analytic encounter, and this emphasises the forgotten (or suppressed) subjectivity of the analyst, understandably an important value when struggling to move away from the deterministic drive theory model. In fact, instead of countertransference, the term 'intersubjectivity' is widely used as something like a synonym. This approach took a view of the analytic relationship as developing a characteristic form, and atmosphere or culture, which is uniquely contributed to by both parties in a democratic manner. It resembles the earlier views of the Balints (1939) as the notion of the 'essential feature'[7], and has been, in part, responsible for the rehabilitation of Balint's mentor, Ferenczi.

---

7 To remind the reader – his essential feature, as described in the quote previously, is 'all these phenomena happen in an inter-relation between two individuals, in a constantly changing and developing object-relation' (1950, p. 123).

Following Balint particularly, the notion of authenticity implies that the analyst has a personality as much as the patient, and the shape and outcome of an analytic treatment will be determined by the input of the analyst's personality as much as the patient's. Whilst it seems merely common sense, the influence of the analyst as a person seems easily forgotten, perhaps because it is professionally uncomfortable to accept that the analyst's own oddities and foibles will add distinctive features to the outcome for the patient's personality.

Social construction/post-modernism: The co-constructivists tend to accept social constructionism, that is, a kind of collaborative idealism – the ideas of both parties collaborate in constructing the culture of the particular analysis. Their ideals, beliefs, and attitudes arise in the interactive network of their communications, and are laid down in their communicative system. This collaborative establishing of what is believed, and ultimately what is seen, can be called co-construction within the psychoanalytic setting of two. From a psychoanalytic point of view, there is no objectivity. What is important is the way the self and others collaborate. Leaving objectivity on one side means that what is observed is the product of pure subjectivity, as it were. The partners construct a unique entity between them. More than an interaction, there is a unified whole, comparable to Balint's (1950) essential feature (see Chapter 5). It is predicated on the assumption that objectivity is unattainable, and, in fact, in a science of subjectivity like psychoanalysis, it may be undesirable.

Field theory: Since the nineteenth century, Gestalt theory was an important theoretical force in European psychology, and it influenced psychoanalysis to some extent. It arrived in the US via Kurt Lewin and his field theory of group dynamics, though more significant in South America (through the Barangers), emigrating from Paris where they learned Gestalt field theory from Merleau-Ponty. Baranger and Baranger (2008) began to understand the analytic encounter in terms of a field, which fits in with the attractive aspects of Ferenczi, and the work of Balint. Jointly, the two parties create a separate entity that sits between them. This has been developed in various directions, as we shall see.

The analytic third: Arising in parallel is an alternative but prominent view of intersubjectivity as a remarkable achievement of the psychoanalytic partners, a third object is created. Perhaps influenced by field theory, the two subjectivities appear to be three, in a very concrete way. This 'analytic third' has been pioneered by Thomas Ogden:

> Over the past several years, I have developed a conception of the analytic process that is based on the idea that in addition to the analyst and analysand, there is a third subject of analysis to which I have referred

as 'the intersubjective analytic third' (Ogden, 1996, p. 884).

He characterised the two partners as each influencing and being influenced by the third object: 'I believe that in an analytic context, there is no such thing as an analysand apart from the relationship with the analyst, and no such thing as an analyst apart from the relationship with the analysand' (Ogden, 2004, p. 168). He acknowledged his debt to Winnicott:

> My own conception of analytic intersubjectivity represents an elaboration and extension of Winnicott's (1960) notion that "there is no such thing as an infant [separate from the maternal provision]" (Ogden, 2004, p. 168).

Ogden is referring to this combined product of subjectivities as a created 'third subjectivity' (Ogden, 1994, p. 64). This position addresses the relationship in a holistic manner rather than picking off the individuals separately. It connects with, and sought support from, Winnicott and his descriptions of a third area, the transitional space, which is specified as having the paradoxical qualities of both 'me' and 'not-me' at the same time. This is the area in which the person can continue to indulge in a form of play (Winnicott, 1971) that gratifies their infantile omnipotence into adult life. Ogden emphasised:

> To summarise briefly the ideas presented in those publications, the intersubjective analytic third is understood as a third subject created by the unconscious interplay of analyst and analysand; at the same time, the analyst and analysand *qua* analyst and analysand are generated in the act of creating the analytic third. (There is no analyst, no analysand, no analysis, aside from the process through which the analytic third is generated.) (Ogden, 1995, p. 697)

There is no equivocation about this – intersubjectivity is a third object. In one of the earliest statements that Ogden makes on intersubjectivity, in 1994, he regarded the object created by the intersubjective collaboration of two people as *the* fact to be discovered by a psychoanalysis (Ogden, 1994).

Ogden's illustration: He gives a clinical case study in his book, *Subjects of Analysis*, to illustrate that objectification (Ogden, 1994). It is beautifully illustrative of the kind of clinical thinking in which Ogden uses his felt experience.

The patient who had been in analysis for some years was tedious to listen to, as he was very distant from his own lively feelings. The analyst, Ogden, was constantly distracted; on one occasion, he noticed an envelope on his desk. He had used the envelope for making some *aide de memoire* notes. But in this session he noticed it anew, for the first time as it were. As he said, 'despite the fact that the envelope had been physically present for weeks, it came to life at that point as a psychological event, a carrier of psychological meanings' (Ogden, 1994, pp. 74-75).

There were a number of aspects that suddenly had emotional significance – it had contained a personal letter, but appeared to be part of a bulk mailing, the stamps were bright and engaging, so was it falsely personal after all, then the address was printed by typewriter, and so must have been personal. The point that Ogden is getting at is not to tell us about the patient so much as his engagement with the envelope at the time he is with the patient. The envelope's new meaning for the analyst was in that specific context. Thus, the 'new' envelope, which he saw for the first time, must have been created in part by the patient being in the room at the time of the analyst's new perception. Therefore, he says the envelope – as experienced – was a creation of *both* parties. The significance in this analysis is that the issues of authenticity about the envelope, which Ogden found worrying in his own mind, are rather strikingly connected with the patient's inauthentic way of talking. However, it is the precise way in which that pressed in on the analyst through the new perception of a third object in the consulting room, which Ogden wants us to recognise with him.

Via the envelope, the analyst is engaged with the patient in co-constructing this new object, a concrete manifestation of their intersubjectivity. Ogden says there is a specificity here. The envelope is seen as new because of the intersubjective dialectic between the analyst and analysand right *now*; 'No thought, feeling, or sensation can be considered to be the same as it was or will be outside of the context of the specific (and continually shifting) intersubjectivity created by analyst and analysand' (Ogden, 1994b, pp. 73-74).

Ogden attributes a subjectivity to the envelope itself, a third subjectivity in the room. This is radical indeed. Whilst most intersubjectivists are not so radical, a contrast with the intra-psychic approach is in high relief. In one approach, the subjectivities are interacting (intra-psychic), and, in the other, the field is co-created by the subjectivities (co-constructivist), which are themselves in continual emergence.

Ogden's 'intersubjective resonance of unconscious processes of individuals experiencing one another as subjects' (1988, p. 23) has created a specific framework for thinking how the patient and analyst, as interdependent subject and object (transference and countertransference), come together to form a 'third object' – or the jointly created analytic third (Ogden, 1994). The analyst's experience, termed the countertransference in its broadest sense, contributes a body of 'intersubjective' clinical facts. He may experience them as the apparently self-absorbed ramblings of his mind, bodily sensations that seemingly have nothing to do with the analysand, or any other intersubjectively generated phenomenon within the analytic pair (Ogden, 1994). It must be true that the analyst, like anyone else, is functioning and experiencing in the moment and in whatever context he is in – including the room in which he is closeted with this specific patient at the appointed time. The context for any analyst at work is the patient he is with. Of course, he brings aspects of himself to bear on the meanings of the context. The therapeutic stress is placed on the fact that the subjectivity of an individual arises out of the intersubjective context of the moment.

This has brought back a re-examination of Sullivan and the long tradition of interpersonal psychoanalysis (Levenson, 1984; Cushman, 1994). However, the therapeutic focus of the intersubjectivists is on the psychoanalytic context, the patient's context being the interacting analyst – and this contrasts with the approach of the earlier Sullivanian interpersonalists who emphasised the social contexts outside the analysis. So, the co-constructivists' focus of interpretation is on the here-and-now, which brings these analysts close to the British schools, although from a different starting point.

Privileging the patient: From a different angle, the failure of objectivity in psychoanalysis is regarded as requiring a radical solution. The psychoanalyst's point of view is far too corrupted by his own irreducible subjectivity, and in consequence the patient's own subjectivity, *their* point of view, is privileged instead of the psychoanalyst's, which is eliminated. This follows the classical psychoanalytic warning about countertransference, but turns away from the 'scientific' technique of the blank-screen analyst who exclusively makes objective observation; instead the blank screen is regarded as impossible and to be abandoned. Schwaber (1996), in reaction to the prevailing privileging of the analyst's point of view, emphasised that the patient's subjectivity must be the one to shine through. Similarly, Kohut's (1971) notion of empathic immersion, endorsed by subsequent self-psychologists, has also led to privileging the patient's point of view.

Owen Renik, debating the prioritisation of the patient, relied on an extreme respect for post-modernism. This strategy leads away from a sense of a nuclear problem to be revealed, a core truth into which we must gain insight, and instead substitutes the capacity to develop intersubjective engagement just for its own sake (e.g. Renik, 1993b). This is a tradition that moves with velocity away from the medical model of pathologising the patient, and its method of fitting patients to the theories of pathology. There is no objective nuclear problem. The patient's point of view has equal (or more) validity than the psychoanalyst's. It paints a picture of two points of view, each fluidly reacting in a negotiating process.

Renik's approach gave rise to a debate based on perspectivism, between himself and Marcia Cavell (in the issues of the *International Journal* in 1998-9; Cavell 1998a, 1998b, 1999; Renik 1998, 1999). Cavell was anxious that Renik's extreme post-modernism, leaves us with nothing but a shifting sand of personal impressions (see the next chapter for details of this debate). At its extreme, the notion of countertransference has been absorbed simply into a consideration of personal style that collaborates with the patient's.

Emerging strands of development

For reasons touched on, the new ideas about countertransference, and therefore of the subjectivity of the psychoanalyst, took longer to take root in North American psychoanalysis than the more intra-psychic object-relations approach. Hence, the two geographical regions present two different conceptual backgrounds deriving from their differing histories. However, this neat geographical division is not in fact so exact. Some British analysts of the Independent tradition have been strongly influenced by the newer developments in America, Ogden's work, the intersubjectivists and relational psychoanalysis, whilst those developments in the US had already been inspired by, and then blended with, the ideas of some British analysts, notably Donald Winnicott. A variant of the post-modernist dissolution of reality into a dream-like shimmer (termed 'waking dreaming' after Bion's 'reverie') has evolved in Italy (Ferro, 2005; Civitarese, 2008).

Moreover, each strand of development is not entirely coherent. As will be apparent, the difference is between a realist approach (generally the intrapsychic), and an idealist one (the co-constructivist). The development of these two main strands has been a complex process, and is not a simple transition from suspicion to useful tool – from bad to good. Warren Poland (2000), in an attempt to capture the new developments, wrote:

> Intersubjectivity used this way, to speak of an interaction, refers to the communicative emotional flow between two different [intra-psychic] parties. This use of intersubjectivity is different from its use to carry a contrary meaning, that of a unified field. In this second sense the word refers to the clinical universe as an intact whole, one in which experience is generated and created by the engaged pair as an essential unity, a singular dyad (Poland, 2000, p. 29).

This bifurcation of the two trends in conceptualising countertransference hits the mark. There is either a complex of two open systems, the intrapsychic approach, or an essentially unified field, a singular dyad. Despite various originating factors we have run through, influencing in varying proportion any psychoanalyst's personal point of view, the two domains

Poland abstracted do mark out the overall geography:

- A complex process deriving from more traditional sources, which can be thought of as an unconsciously negotiated dramatisation of two subjectivities. This is the intrapsychic approach to countertransference, where something real in the other is assumed.

- The democratising and authentic process in which the analyst's feelings, as a person, are included as a balancing manoeuvre to equate with the patient's feelings, and described as creating a unified 'field' co-constructed by the personality characteristics of both partners.

Despite this attempt to clarify the distinctions, perhaps it is the case at present that there would be difficulty in mapping out a coherent plan of the different developmental trajectories, and we might even make up a few more classifications. As indicated in this book, the main developments arise, roughly speaking, from two different originating historical and conceptual sources – one the contemporary views of countertransference arising from an object-relations focus, the other those developments that are superseding ego-psychology.

Added in is the classical view, which seems to be clearly declining in the present and over the recent past, which still holds countertransference under suspicion, and believes that intersubjectivity dangerously flouts objectivity.

CHAPTER 8

Critical debate – Conclusions to Part 2
How do the trends compare?

The intra-psychic object-relations point of view, and the co-constructive intersubjectivist point of view, have now lifted the weight of suspicion on countertransference, and have diverged into two main trends – each with its fundamentally specific set of assumptions. One trend, the intrapsychic, has a realist assumption that there is a real other who is knowable. In some respects, at least the analyst can know something about his patients, and their experiences. In contrast, the co-constructivist assumption is an idealist one; the patient is a creation of the analyst's experience of him, and vice versa, an interaction that has no reality outside the fragile moment of meeting in each psychoanalytic session. These fundamental differences between a belief in a real knowable other, and the other as a construction, are clear-cut. In natural science, these complexities don't really exist, but when the object of study is another mind, the sets of assumptions and their differences are far from clear, and I am not going to examine these complex differences here. However, each approach naturally has criticisms of the other.

The co-constructive approach started out from a critique of classical psychoanalysis as it had survived as ego-psychology and drive theory. Though the intra-psychic position is not at all identical with classical psychoanalysis, some of the founding criticism from the co-constructivist position does apply to the more objective and even 'scientific' intra-psychic position. The significant critiques by the co-constructive position of the intra-psychic positions fall into several categories:

- the privileging of the psychoanalyst, with the power imbalance implied;

- the subjectivity of the analyst;

- the need to take account of the intersubjective social construction (post-modern influence);

- the refocused attention of the psychoanalyst.

In turn, the intra-psychic adherents can respond with critiques of the co-constructive position:

- the ultra relativism;

- intersubjective constructions instead of knowledge (throwing the baby of reality out with the bathwater);

- hidden privileging.

Constructing a mutual critique

Under several headings, I will attempt to convey the debate that might be had currently between the core members of each tradition.

Objective reality and subjectivity. This intra-psychic claim that the analyst's subjectivity can have an objective reference point is regarded dubiously by the co-constructivists, for whom the reality in psychoanalysis is undeniably subjective. The relative roles of subjectivity and objectivity do not and cannot conform to those of natural science, despite Freud's claims.

From this point of view, the intra-psychic position claims a privileged place for the analyst's objectivity on the patient's subjectivity. Renik argued that the analyst is himself 'irreducibly subjective' (Renik, 1993b, p. 562). The analyst's point of view on the patient's point of view will inevitably be so corrupted by the analyst's subjectivity that it should be seriously questioned, and left aside in favour of the patient's account of his experiences. So, we need to re-focus our attention from an objective claim by either (i) privileging the patient's subjectivity, or (ii) analysing the analytic third.

In the intra-psychic approach, there is not such an acceptance of the purely post-modern, social construction of reality. The clinical material speaks, at least in part, objectively, demanding a classical respect for the substance of the patient's material. The dream, for instance, is from the beginning of psychoanalysis the *object* of study.

Co-constructivism can seem extreme in this respect. How far should the criticism of the analyst's subjective position be taken? Dunn protested that 'the irreducibility of our subjectivity does not reduce us to total ignorance' (Dunn, 1995, p. 723). Also, 'Evidence that the analyst knows something that the patient does not know is welcome to most patients. If it were not, why would anyone pay for analysis?' (Richards and Richards, 1995, p. 442) – a hard-nosed view that might be tricky to answer from the co-constructive position.

Kantian reality: The concern about privileged objective knowing that led to this turn towards a post-modern view can imply any knowledge is purely a point of view, ultimately unreliable and evanescent. The position is rightly a Kantian one, where we can only know things as filtered through *a priori* expectations built into the subjectivity of human understanding – the subjectivity of space, time and causality (according to Kant). So instead, co-constructivism variously adopts a social constructivism, a mutuality, an intersubjectivity and a perspectivism.

Marcia Cavell (1998a, 1998b, 1999), a philosophically knowledgeable psychoanalyst, reacted to the extreme relativism of Owen Renik (1998, 1999) with the view that there must be some generalities to be had from the encounter between analyst and patient, however subjective each partner is. Her intermediate position – between simply privileging the patient's subjectivity, and acting on the authority of the psychoanalyst – can be called a perspectivism. She pointed out that even the material external world can be seen differently by people who have different interests. Her example is an astronomer who looks at the stars in a different way from a hiker who wants to find his way. The astronomer sees the earth rotating, whilst the hiker views the stars as rotating; these are entirely sufficient for each of their two purposes. Two people observing from different perspectives see things differently, but they see the *same thing* differently.

Because there are two (or more) points of view on an occurrence, it does not rule out an objective reality. Recognising that things are always seen from a perspective does not stop us saying some entity out-there can still be said to exist. It could still be the object of study, even if we have only a perspective on it. In a sense, reality is always unknown, insofar as it is not *completely* known.

Kant was actually referring to natural science and the approximation and relativism of knowledge of the material world. He described the thing-in-itself, a full knowledge of a material object cannot be known, but some knowledge of it can be, and even partial knowledge is useful. The hiker does not need to know the debate between Ptolemy and Copernicus, only how the stars are positioned, and how far they appear to have moved in a given time period. Is it any different for psychoanalytic knowledge? If we grant that we will never know everything about a patient's subjective experience, it is still possible that we can know something – and that something can be psychoanalytically useful. Thus, the critique is that the patient's mind is only an object of psychoanalytic study when we observe things relevant for psychoanalytic work. That is a perspectivism; the perspective we view it from must be relevant for what we want to do with the knowledge.

Having different perspectives contributes a two-sided description, or triangulation borrowing from the technology, and mathematics of surveying. Cavell developed a kind of triangulation of the patient's mind – a view from inside the patient, and a view from outside, the psychoanalyst's – which gives the possibility of some integration, and more reliable knowledge than either alone. One could say a subjective component, from the psychoanalyst's feelings, meets an objective component, the contents of the associations by the patient. That recommendation echoes Heimann's (1960) similar triangulation of perspectives – the countertransference and the actual material of the session, though Cavell did not make the connection with Heimann.

Who decides: Odgen's mutually constructed subjective third aims to give an even-handedness to the influence of the partners, avoiding privileging either. *Both* co-construct together, delivering an intersubjectivity. The countertransference is then rescued, after the fashion Cavell suggested, by balancing the analyst's subjectivity with the patient's. At the same time, there is a difficulty in these descriptions; it is difficult to avoid wondering who it is who decides what the third object is – in Ogden's example it was the psychoanalyst who found the envelope in his mind, and we do not hear if that object is a construct in the patient's mind as well. It seems unlikely. Whilst on the one hand the aim is to 'democratise' the setting, as it were, there is also a tendency to revert to prioritising the analyst's decision about what the 'third object' is.

The apparent egalitarian intention may be more apparent than real. Whose perspective on the field counts? And how is it made to count? It is also a problem for the co-constructivist view that, as Freud originally noted, the interactive process is unconscious and inherently unknown consciously. Much of the move towards a field theory of the third object is the inadvertent privileging of consciousness, and the risk then of slipping into a form of systems theory that side-lines the dynamic unconscious.

If so, then Orange (1995) puzzled, 'at times [analysts] can be so involved in and devoted to getting and staying close to the patient's experience that we may forget that we are there too' (Orange, 1995, p. 66). However, Hanly makes a philosophical distinction:

> One could agree that the analyst, like any person, can be correctly characterized as irreducibly subjective in the psychological and moral senses of the term, without agreeing that analysts are irreducibly subjectivist in the epistemological sense (Hanly and Hanly, 2001, p. 518).

Glen Gabbard (1997) also argued against the post-modern privileging of the patient's subjectivity, on the grounds that the analyst is surely there for some reason. His common-sense point is that the analyst's advantage is that he sees the patient's point of view *from another* point of view. Thus, a perspectivist approach to the problem of objectivity can be usefully developed and used.

Power and privilege: First, from the co-constructivist viewpoint, the intrapsychic perspective appears to see the patient as a real, other subject, knowable – and also influenceable – by the subjectivity of the psychoanalyst. He privileges his own claims to know the subjectivity of the analysand over the patient's knowledge.

The philosopher Thomas Nagel (1987) called this a 'view from nowhere', above the battlefield, as it were. It assumes the analyst's subjectivity is immune (relatively) from the distortions that make the patient's subjectivity so unreliable and vulnerable to unconscious and extraneous influences. So, in the intrapsychic approach, the psychoanalyst risks being all-knowing about the subjectivity of the other.

The question is whether it is at all possible to eliminate some degree of privileging of the psychoanalyst. There seems to be a loop that is hard to escape – while trying to establish a mutually constructed 'third' in the room, the analyst is helplessly thrown back into the role of being the one who decides what it is.

A privileged objectivity is risky since it can inform action, giving psychoanalysts power to intrude and mould the development of the patient; a Foucauldian criticism, based on the view that knowledge is power. At its worst, it is the wielding of pre-existing theory over the ephemeral and fragile moment of experience – the deadening hand of theory.

Field (intermingling): It may be argued by the co-constructivist positon that the subjective intermingling of two minds cannot be ignored. The creation of that subjective field is, in practice, quite different from the objective science of the material world where there is real separation of objects and influences. From the intra-psychic position, however, it can be acknowledged that the two intrapsychic worlds may well become seriously intermingled and confused, but there is still a clue to the actual contributions from both sides, in the process and the meaningful content of the clinical material. Disentangling the field may therefore privilege the analyst's view (or even the patient's unconscious view) and may push away the patient's creativity and play.

Shallow/consciousness. Then, it is argued, we must arrange the setting to be a mutuality, and be respectful of the intersubjective perspectives. Such an approach was held up to view in an Editorial to the *Journal of the American Psychoanalytic Association*, 'The current era is not without critics who point out its tendencies toward relativism, pastiche, and nostalgia' (Litowitz, 2002, p. 17).

Similarly, without the advantage of objectivity, can it be argued that only the patient's point of view about his own point of view is sufficient? Against that view, we can query what the analyst adds, for his professional fee.

Summary of assumptions

This debate has evolved, it seems, into a set of assumptions underlying each approach, which can be systematised roughly:

- Aims
    - For the co-constructivists, the assumption is that the partners enter a joint creativity, joining them with each other in a kind of playful union with free

expression of drives in a non-coercive relational context.

o The intra-psychic approach, in contrast, sticks to the traditional interpretation of communications from the unconscious, such as dreams, and the transference and the countertransference experience.

- Intervention

  o For the co-constructivist approach, it appears to be a process of practice learning for an authentic relating that balances self-determination with attunement with each other.

  o However, for the intra-psychic approach, the intervention resolves the level of anxiety that drives the defences, symptoms, and relationship disorders, and allows development under the dominance of the reality principle.

- Results

  o The co-constructivist result will be a step up in lively authentic relating, measured by the attainment of personal goals.

  o For the intra-psychic approach, there will be an

increased level of maturity in handling anxieties, and relating less defensively or intrusively with others.

- The privileged authority of the psychoanalyst

  o The co-constructivist analyst still decides the level of authenticity, for instance, what the 'third object' is, whilst also avowedly promoting a respect for the patient's perspective.

  o In the intra-psychic approach, the analyst privileges his own assessment of the patient's response to interpretation (response to insight) – not his own response to the interpretation.

This is a preliminary categorisation of initial assumptions of the two approaches. It is a schema that would benefit from a formal research project.

Conclusion: An elephant in the room

An argument of a perspectivist kind arises in ancient sources going back to the Buddha, to whom is attributed the parable of the 'Blind men and the elephant' (see Epilogue to this chapter). The parable briefly is that six blind men observe an elephant – by touching it. One interprets the leg as a tree, one the tail as a rope, one the body as a wall, and so on. The implication is that those viewing from different perspectives interpret the same thing differently. It is a view Bion (with an Indian heritage himself, though he never mentioned the ancient parable) turned into a book-length argument about the mathematical idea of transformations (Bion, 1965). His target was not countertransference, but the general plethora of unintegrated theories that make up psychoanalytic metapsychology. For instance, he started his book like this:

> Suppose a painter sees a path through a field sown with poppies and paints it: at one end of the chain of events is the field of poppies, at the other a canvas with pigment disposed on its surface. We can recognize that the latter represents the former, so I shall suppose that despite the differences between a field of poppies and a piece of canvas, despite the transformation that the artist has effected in what he saw to make it take the form of a picture, something has remained unaltered and on this something recognition depends (Bion, 1965, p. 1).

There is something out there that has a correspondence resonating in all the differing recognitions. There is a commonality in the various correspondences. That commonality in the variance, however minimal, he called the 'invariant'. Bion's target was to promote investigation of what are the common invariants between patient and analyst, and, importantly, between one psychoanalytic school and another.

This is one of Bion's most Kantian statements, and like Cavell's about the astronomer and the hiker, it represents the difference of perspective according to one's purpose. The nature of countertransference is similarly various according to the two purposes of the intrapsychic and the co-constructivist trends. On the one hand, the purpose was to begin a conceptualisation of the clinical process of intra-psychic relating between analyst and patient, both parties being in fact persons making relations. On the other hand, the co-constructivists' purpose was to find a more personal view of the relationship than drive theory could yield, whilst in a culture of progressively rhetorical social equality. There is in both trends some degree of decentring the pathology from the patient, and an analytic humility about the performance of the analyst. However, the emphasis is different, with the tendency to downplay pathology itself in the intra-psychic approach and to investigate the interactive process between the disturbances of the two parties. Amongst the co-constructivists, there is a more strongly held sense that the analyst should shoulder a large share of the responsibility and culpability for their disturbance then the patient.

Epilogue to Chapter 8

THE BLIND MEN AND THE ELEPHANT

(The version of the famous Indian legend attributed to the Buddha, but rendered wittily by the American Poet – available, July 2016, at http://www.noogenesis.com/pineapple/blind_men_elephant.html –)

John Godfrey Saxe (1816-1887)

It was six men of Indostan

To learning much inclined,

Who went to see the Elephant

(Though all of them were blind),

That each by observation

Might satisfy his mind.

The First approach'd the Elephant,

And happening to fall

Against his broad and sturdy side,

At once began to bawl:

"God bless me! but the Elephant

Is very like a wall!"

The Second, feeling of the tusk,

Cried, -"Ho! what have we here

So very round and smooth and sharp?

To me 'tis mighty clear

This wonder of an Elephant

Is very like a spear!"

The Third approached the animal,

And happening to take

The squirming trunk within his hands,

Thus boldly up and spake:

"I see," quoth he, "the Elephant

Is very like a snake!"

The Fourth reached out his eager hand,

And felt about the knee.

"What most this wondrous beast is like

Is mighty plain," quoth he,

"'Tis clear enough the Elephant

Is very like a tree!"

The Fifth, who chanced to touch the ear,

Said: "E'en the blindest man

Can tell what this resembles most;

Deny the fact who can,

This marvel of an Elephant

Is very like a fan!"

The Sixth no sooner had begun

About the beast to grope,

Then, seizing on the swinging tail

That fell within his scope,

"I see," quoth he, "the Elephant

Is very like a rope!"

And so these men of Indostan

Disputed loud and long,

Each in his own opinion

Exceeding stiff and strong,

Though each was partly in the right,

And all were in the wrong!

MORAL.

So oft in theologic wars,

The disputants, I ween,

Rail on in utter ignorance

Of what each other mean,

And prate about an Elephant

Not one of them has seen!

CHAPTER 9

Interlude – The unconscious in Freud
Can we test the new view?

Much of Freud's detailed clinical notes in his classic cases remains available – notably Little Hans and the Rat Man – and can be investigated for traces of the processes not then recognised. If we examine for, and find, emotional traces of countertransference in its modern sense, then it is likely that the modern conception is not just an artefact of our theories, or of our contemporary assumptions, but is deeply inherent in the psychoanalytic process itself. Previously, I showed (Hinshelwood, 2013b) that three of Freud's case reports (the Wolf Man, the Rat Man, and Little Hans) did indeed reveal elements of our contemporary understanding of transference, countertransference, and enactment. Reviews of these phenomena occurring in Freud's case material have occasionally been reported (Mahoney, 1984, 1986; Etchegoyen, 1988; Gottlieb, 1989; Hinshelwood, 1989; Rudnytsky, 1999; Blum, 2007) – but little discussed.

Here I shall merely summarise what can be gleaned from the literature, using two of the cases – the Rat Man and the Wolf

Man. What I shall indicate is a process in which the analyst, Freud, is clearly moved by emotions arising in the moment of a session. He responded in active ways. At the time, technique was not as strictly bounded as now, so that going outside the role as now conceived is more obvious, and shows more transparently the pressure on the analyst. Thus, it is quite possible to see how the analyst is moved, and responds actively to unconscious determinants in the process of his interaction.

To identify these moments where countertransference appears, I shall use three characteristics:

- The patient's transference;

- Indications of the psychoanalyst's emotional responses expressed indirectly (the countertransference);

- Some untoward enactment by the analyst, out-of-role, but unconsciously appropriate to his or her emotional state.

The Rat Man

Freud wrote up the analysis of Ernst Lanzer, the 'Rat Man' (Freud, 1909a), for the purpose of extending theory. This patient gave him the chance to demonstrate intense unmodified aggression and sadism in obsessional patients, which he had postulated earlier (Freud, 1894). Freud recognised that the obsessional felt his imagination had real consequences – 'the omnipotence of phantasy' (Freud, 1909a, p. 233).

Freud left process notes of the case (published by Strachey in the *Standard Edition*), and one identifiable moment of countertransference occurs in the text of the paper, on pages 166–167, and in the Notes on pages 280–282.

The patient's transference: Freud's impression was of someone in a confessional, but who also felt a resistance to telling Freud. Freud thought:

> [It was like an] element of revenge against me... [I] had shown him that by refusing to tell me and by giving up the treatment he would be taking a more outright revenge on me than by telling me (p. 281).

The immediate transference was therefore a rather cruel intention, and Freud was aware of this as a negative transference with its anal-sadistic roots in an obsessional patient. But, the Rat Man, however, felt in great pain at what he inflicted on others:

> At all the more important moments while he was telling his story his face took on a very strange, composite expression. I could only interpret it as one of horror at pleasure of his own of which he himself was unaware. (pp. 166–167)

So the transference was constructed as an ambivalent conflict between his revenge and his exquisitely regretful confession.

The analyst's emotional reactions: In reaction to this transference, Freud felt some sympathy, and was moved by the patient's anguish. However, Freud also said, 'At that moment the idea flashed through my mind that this was happening to a person who was very dear to me.' (p. 167). And even more alarming, Freud wrote in his clinical Notes, 'only after this did he give me to understand that it concerned my daughter' (p. 281). Freud's reaction is implicit in the Notes; but the patient expressed it more explicitly when the patient said that Freud's interpretations 'looked like anxiety on [Freud's] part' (p. 281). So, the alarm in the countertransference is evidenced by the patient's observation.

This arousal of anxiety in Freud may also be a version of a sadistic intrusion in the transference-countertransference, which was being re-enacted at the level of a psychological intrusion into Freud's peace of mind.

Some untoward and unconscious action of the analyst: Freud did not interpret the immediate here-and-now transference – the patient's cruel intrusion of anxiety. Rather, Freud engaged in a more active way, in fact acting out his anxiety. It led him forcefully to prompt the confessional, or perhaps to engage in a 'counter-intrusion':

I went on to say that I would do all I could, nevertheless, to guess the full meaning of any hints he gave me. Was he perhaps thinking of impalement? – "No, not that; . . . the criminal was tied up . . ." – he expressed himself so indistinctly that I could not immediately guess in what position – " . . . a pot was turned upside down on his buttocks . . . some rats were put into it . . . and they . . . " – he had again got up, and was showing every sign of horror and resistance – "… bored their way in . . ." – Into his anus, I helped him out (p. 166).

The point is that the record indicates how Freud was impelled by his own strong feelings. Now we would understand it as an anxious countertransference that led Freud actively to push the patient to divulge his secrets.

Here, Freud appears to give evidence of his intrusions into the patient's mind, and the implicit acting out together of the Rat Man's sadomasochistic phantasy, albeit in a psychic modality. Freud displays in the way he writes (but also apparently even during the sessions with the Rat Man) a certain state of mind that is referred to by the patient as anxious. His manner and behaviour suggest that he is strongly moved by conflict and alarm, to react in line with the patient's problems. The content of the problem, and the process of the analytic encounter, appear to converge into a common triangulated narrative, a narrative about intrusion. We can say that the countertransference can be read from this, together with its motivating power.

The Wolf Man

Like the Rat Man, Freud used the Wolf Man case to report theoretical advances. The Wolf Man (Sergei Pankejeff) was treated in 1913–1914, at the time when Freud was writing his comprehensive papers on metapsychology. Published in 1918, Freud described for the first time the childhood phantasy of the primal scene.

The patient's transference: Freud conveyed how from the beginning to the end of treatment, the Wolf Man remained extremely passive. Freud wrote:

> The patient with whom I am here concerned remained for a long time unassailably entrenched behind an attitude of obliging apathy (Freud, 1918, p. 11)

Freud found the passivity of the patient powerful, it seems. The patient appeared to want Freud to find the way to do the work.

The analyst's emotional state: Freud's choice of phrase is revealing – 'unassailably entrenched' and 'obliging apathy' – and conveys quite a strong response to the patient. Freud is not complimentary. We can infer he was exasperated by the passivity. Freud continued in the same emotive way:

> His shrinking from a self-sufficient existence was so great as to outweigh all the vexations of his illness. (Freud, 1918, p. 11)

Here, this form of expression points to the writer's frustration and even boredom. Despite translation from the German, Freud's writing is very expressive of his personal responses.

Some untoward and unconscious action of the analyst: Freud, in some sort of desperation to change things, seemed to feel compelled to do something (to be the active one). The Wolf Man's 'shrinking' from the necessary developmental process, led Freud to think:

> Only one way was to be found of overcoming it. I was obliged to wait until his attachment to myself had become strong enough to counter-balance this shrinking, and then played off this one factor against the other. (Freud, 1918, p. 11)

Freud had to overcome the resistance, and his impatience led him to set a date for ending the analysis. Freud was both actively challenging the resistance, and also, potentially, putting an end to his own frustration. He had been provoked into reacting actively to the patient's passivity.

Once again, the words chosen, and the attitudes, demonstrate a state of mind and feelings of the analyst, which interestingly co-ordinated precisely with how he conducted himself with the patient. He appears motivated by unconscious intent, not least to relieve his own feelings of frustration. The conditions of a countertransference expressed in words and actions appears in the Wolf Man case, as well as the Ratman.

The archaeology of countertransference

This is almost archaeological evidence from the past. Countertransference as it is conceived today, following the paradigm shift, can be identified by three key characteristics (transference, countertransference, and what we now call an enactment). These features can be spotted in material from the past when countertransference was on the whole viewed with deep suspicion, and avowedly dealt with by suppression and a thick skin. Freud clearly failed to thicken his skin enough, and remained an ordinary enough human being in an ordinary encounter with at least two of his patients. So the wider view of countertransference, as the general reactiveness of the analyst, and an unconscious call to action, did occur visibly even within the less strict technique a century ago. Not until our contemporary understanding could the phenomena have been described or understood. So, these long ago records are a retrospective verification of our understanding.

These unintended details in the records give us compelling support for the wider view of countertransference. The analyst, despite his own advice, was moved to emotional responses that amounted to significant action. These moments seem to come alive in a way, but concealed under the cloak of persistent intellectual and clinical investigation. Perhaps that concealing is the nature of the 'thick skin' that Freud advised.

PART 3

AT WORK TODAY

Today's debates about countertransference, of whatever form, have gradually turned in favour of Heimann's position; that is, we can know a lot about the patient from examining ourselves. The precise method of knowledge generation in the clinical setting is not a settled question. Despite Heimann's move away from Klein, the Klein group has had the longest experience of developing the ideas and the clinical approach towards countertransference. Some of the more enthusiastic of the first protagonists were Klein's followers. They had the advantage of a specific concept of Klein's, the primitive mechanism of projective identification.

Part 3 of this book will concentrate on these developments as they stand today. The conceptualisation of roles redistributed as transference and countertransference emerges more and more as a form of narrative, a narrative enacted in the analytic setting. Countertransference is therefore an attention to process. As such, it marks a distinct step away from the thematic analysis of the *content* of dreams, as used by Freud.

We will consider some problems posed by patients today, the

so-called hard-to-reach patients. They often have a problem with treatment itself as the core issue, and set out to defeat the psychoanalyst for one reason or other. Characteristically, they employ a method of resistance that incorporates the analyst himself, and his feelings, in a role that assists resisting. One of the most prominent contemporary developments in understanding this kind of resistance has been the work of Betty Joseph (1989; Hargreaves and Varchevker, 2004). She exhaustively followed the *micro*-process in sessions as the patient nudged the analyst (often willingly) into enactments.

The joint unconscious enactments are often very difficult for the analyst to spot. The four chapters that follow will exemplify how the analyst is himself playing a role. Simply by being interested, he can implicate himself in a defence the patient employs. This kind of 'use' of the analyst's own personality can be troubling for him, and the patient may then be confronted by a defensive analyst. These chapters recognise that, inevitably, patient and analyst are at cross-purposes, in part at least and sometimes wholly, when the patient doubts the analyst can face the intolerable experiences the patient cannot himself tolerate. Then the situation is such that on one hand, the analyst thinks he is helping the patient to gain insight, whilst the patient in surreptitious ways is engaging the analyst in a role that will sustain his defensiveness. If the patient fundamentally believes he needs his defensive protection because insight is too dangerous, then it may prove very difficult for the analyst to understand that they are both 'missing' each other.

CHAPTER 10

Enactment
What's happening?

It is deeply ingrained in the analyst's professional super-ego that he should refrain from all enactment, but, it is almost inevitable. As Feldman says:

> The difficult and often painful task for the analyst is to recognise the subtle and complex enactments he is inevitably drawn into with his patient, and to work to find a domain for understanding and thought outside the narrow and repetitive confines unconsciously demanded by the patient, and sometimes by his own anxieties and needs (Feldman, 1997, p. 235-236).

There are certain key characteristics in this approach summarised by Feldman in this quote. I draw attention to:

- The analyst's task is painful for some reason.

- He is drawn into enacting a role in a complex form of defence.

- The range of understanding is restricted.

- The analyst must seek to expand this domain for understanding.

So, the analyst must keep up a relentless introspection of his feelings, the analyst's post-graduate analysis (as Money-Kyrle called it), or the state of mind Bion called 'reverie'.

In this chapter, we will look at this kind of description of what 'happens' in the analytic session, as opposed to just what is said. This process of interaction troubles not only the professional super-ego, which frowns darkly on such blind collusive interaction, but it is also troubling for the analyst's unconscious insofar as he is often stirred at unconscious levels of anxiety and defences. If – or when – we do find ourselves pressed into actually enacting roles, it is only by reflecting on what we have got ourselves into that we can then understand the patient's side of this, and our own.

Inevitable enacting

This reflective work by the analyst on his own experience can reveal exactly what is to be evaded. Feldman and Spillius wrote of:

> ...the pressure that analysts may feel under to ease the pain, often by some form of activity (such as answering questions, giving reassurance, or giving explanations) whose tacit meaning to the patient is that the analyst

> cannot stand the pain either (Feldman and Spillius, 1989, p. 50).

Then the analyst is provoked towards defensive moves that have the quality of actions – to do something to change the relationship – rather than to articulate the pain of it. To understand the analyst's conflict between managing the painful discomfort that Feldman referred to, and opening a reflective space demands a persisting emphasis on the here-and-now. This clinical challenge has been investigated particularly by Betty Joseph (1989), about whom Feldman and Spillius were commenting.

Let me now give a brief example of an analysis from some years ago, which proved a failure because the understanding that could come from the countertransference was not understood early enough. In fact, only later as I wrote these notes could I speculate on alternatives:

> This patient in his early thirties was in a tedious office job with no prospects. On meeting him I felt a sympathy, even a similarity that I might have originally presented to my own analyst. I wanted to help him take his opportunities. The treatment was three times a week which he could ill afford. During an initial period of some six months he told a little about himself, and about his current life, where he was isolated and

seemed to want to find a more enjoyable existence if only he could. After that his sessions declined into long silences for a period of a couple of years before he left. I increasingly had the impression that I could find little useful to say to him. Nothing seemed to move him. I was learning what a deadening effect can feel like. These silences were not interesting; I didn't find myself curious about what was going on. I was troubled about how much I should engage him by starting a conversation, asking questions, etc., which was very much against my usual view that patients need their own time and space. On the whole I did not initiate discussion – but then felt it was a waste of the little money he had. I felt an obligation to make something successful of his opportunity in therapy. I have not had such a silent patient before, or since.

One day in the middle of a session he told me a dream. This was very unusual and I prepared to make something of the dream that would set the therapy in motion at last. However, the dream was rather empty and not dramatically told. He summarised it in fact.

In the dream it was as if he lived on another planet out in empty space.

He did not give associations, and it felt there could be

no associations to such a bleak dream. But I had an association. At some time, probably within the previous year, a space shuttle had disintegrated on launching. I was not at all sure what to do with the thought. Such bleakness and disaster seemed overwhelming. And I seemed responsible. I am pretty sure he never brought another dream.

For some sessions after this, I remember that I found myself quite pre-occupied with the disaster. At that point I did begin to address what sort of part I was playing in this bleak therapy. What I worked out in my mind was that when I hoped that we could now get going and launch the therapy as it were, nothing in fact happened. I had no idea if the space launch disaster was something he knew about. But I did eventually some time later make an interpretation, saying that it was as if the therapy had not got started, but that we were still waiting, although we seemed to remain out of communication so much. I knew at the time that this could have been taken as somewhat critical, and to my surprise, he actually came to life, getting quite angry. He told me that I was like an empty hole and there was nothing he could expect of me. Thereafter he subsided again. This show of emotion was so unusual that I did remark on it. I said, 'You are disappointed in me, and had hoped for something different from therapy. I think you wanted me to inject some life into the process here, and I have not done so.' He shrugged his shoulders as if hopeless, and after a little silence said in a calm way again, 'It's the dream isn't it?' I thought he was right, so I said, 'Well we are talking about it now, aren't we?", and I think I must have conveyed some hope in my voice. He did not make any movement or say anything, as if anaesthetising things again. But in a few minutes, he said, 'Well, I don't want to disappoint you.'

This therapy was not a success... On reflecting now, I could see that there was something like an aborted take-off, as if hope always crashes down into despair. When for the first and only time he showed some strong lively feeling, his anger, perhaps when he felt criticised, vanished as quickly as it had come. I could say I did reach him, momentarily, and provoked an engaged anger. I did not know how to proceed. It appeared that two things happened; first in my countertransference I found some hope; then, second in the interaction between us, hope was destroyed. The construction I make with hindsight, though there isn't real evidence, is that unconsciously he brought this painful phantasy that always hope must be disappointed, and in the analysis I was supposed to keep it safe, that I should be a shuttle that survived and carried his hope safely. I have always felt sad at not being able to help him more.

I offer this as an example of an enactment of a disastrous take-off – into inner space. The dream led me to hope, and to engage on that basis. A live moment of expectation occurred. I think this was an enactment, as the term is used today. Whilst I listened with all the reverie I could manage, and recognised my frustrations and hopes, my uncertainties about what to do about his silences, coping with the guilt of his wasted money, and so on, I fell into the fatal enactment.

Whilst I was struggling to engage in a process of discovery that could draw some picture of his inner world, he was doing something else. He needed to cope with his belief that hope would be forever dashed. I was used as the mind into which to export the hope (and the disappointment). The analysis was a success from *his* point of view so long as he was spared the feeling of a disappointed hope. That use of me was a conveniently offered opportunity whereby I was given a role that could spare him the intolerable feeling of disappointment. In my experience at the time, I could not gain an awareness of my role so that we could understand together how he protected himself against the disappointments he felt were inevitable and unbearable.

I seemed to succumb to disappointment instead of keeping his hopes alive – a moment that might have offered me occasion for 'a silent piece of self-analysis' as Money-Kyrle recommended. I could really only get the meaning of the experience when he gave the dream and *my* association illuminated it. The enactment is not physical action; it is the 'act' of taking on the hoping (and disappointment). It is an 'emotional act'.

This sad case demonstrates the following key characteristics identified by Feldman in the quote given earlier in the Chapter:

- It is true, the analyst's task was painful; I can attest to that, as I struggled in my uncertainty about how to listen to his silences, and to cope with hopes that are disappointed,

- The second characteristic was how the analyst is drawn into a complex defence. The role assigned to me to enact appeared to be that of carrying the hope; moreover, I was induced into this role by my very act of trying to be an analyst and trying to get the analysis to take off once he told me the dream,

- The next characteristic is the very restricted domain allowed for understanding; and this definitely applied, for the silences (and perhaps the sense of lost curiosity about them) hampered this joint work on what was going on. The patient's comment on not wanting to disappoint me offered only one moment to get some idea of the role assigned to me – i.e. to keep hope alive. In a sense, there was a profound control of my mind and my ability to have my own thoughts, a real problem of separation that I seemed to fall in with in this particular dynamic of ours.

- In the event, I could not find a way to use that leverage, and thus I continued in the role, and enactment – manifesting the abortive mission of the analysis with this patient.

The analyst is not just a role-responding object that fits in with the patient's phantasy world in order to display it. He does fit in with a responsiveness, but each analyst does so in his own way. For instance, there was something about Money-Kyrle's introjection of his patient's feeling of persecuted uselessness that touched the analyst in a specific way (see Chapter 5). It touched, he said, a 'part of the analyst not yet understood'. What is actualised in the analyst is something already there, something the analyst should be expected to identify for himself – silently, Money-Kyrle advised. The patient's projection was not just introjected by the analyst, but it activated some aspect of the analyst that accepted the patient's introjection

(Brenman Pick, 1985).

Joseph's nudging

Rather than finding new theoretical models, Betty Joseph concentrated on the new technique opened by the awareness of countertransference. She was originally analysed by Michael Balint during her training as a psychoanalyst in the 1940s. Subsequently, she had an analysis with Paula Heimann around the time of her the countertransference moment in 1950. Joseph became interested in patients who were 'hard to reach', as she put it. Particular patients seemed to resist analysis, just for the sake of doing so. For Betty Joseph, that resistance has a special quality connected with disturbing their balance of mind, their psychic equilibrium. That balance is one between acknowledging the help, as opposed to a destructive, and self-destructive, twisting of the help into something else. So, these patients are particularly susceptible to change, even to therapeutic change – or, perhaps, especially to therapeutic change. Change risks undoing the equilibrium that the patient has managed to achieve, however unsatisfactorily. He might prefer to endure lifelessness, rather than plunge into a live moment that disturbs him.

There is, it seems, both a defensiveness against insights that arouse conflict and pain, and also a perverse resistant destructiveness against what is beneficial, just for the sake of it. Those two motives are often seen as distinctly different and separate in their operation. It appears as a sort of double resistance, creating the special difficulties an analyst has with these hard-to-reach patients. However, Joseph's attention pointed in a different direction – not the old chestnut whether destructiveness is death instinct or frustrated life instinct (see Chapter 13). Instead, she drew attention to the other discrepancy, as outlined above – whilst the analyst thinks the process is generating insight, the patient thinks the analyst is available for the purpose of strengthening his defences (Hargreaves and Varchevker, 2004).

Patients with these difficult characteristics may come to the psychoanalyst more often now than in the past. They have defeated other forms of therapy by using the therapist for defensiveness, rather than for treatment. Indeed, perhaps those *easy* to reach patients who have more capacity to use treatments for what they actually offer are, in fact, more amenable to simple methods like medication or behavioural therapies, and so achieve enough relief for their purpose. Then again, it may be that we are today looking more precisely for unconscious processes that escaped previous generations of analysts.

The analyst is drawn unwittingly into the patient's difficulty and is recruited to play a role that supports the patient's efforts to defeat insight. The analyst is recruited against himself, and he frequently complies. She wrote:

> [The strategy in,] forcing him [the analyst] into a

> particular role, is a constant process going on in the analytic situation… the analyst is in the mind of the patient drawn into the process, continually being used as a part of his defensive system (Joseph, 1989, p. 126).

For Joseph, this constant process occupies both patient and analyst all the time, so that the whole of an analysis has to be thought of as transference; all the associations are in part a reference, conscious or unconscious, to this immediate transference-countertransference relationship.

The analyst is required to play a central role, that role being defined by a projective identification into the analyst:

> Much of the hatred against parts of the self is now directed towards the mother. This leads to a particular kind of identification which establishes the prototype of an aggressive object relation. I suggest for these processes the term 'projective identification'. When projection is mainly derived from the infant's impulse to harm or to control the mother, he feels her to be a persecutor (Klein, 1952, p. 300-301).

The analyst is required unconsciously to respond by conforming to the role of harmed and controlled mother. It is role-responsiveness (Sandler, 1976). There are implications for the analyst if he is coaxed into the patient's defensive phantasies in the moment he is trying to reveal them. He is puzzled and defeated.

Joseph's emphasis on the here-and-now may not appeal to some, on the grounds that it relegates historical reconstruction to a secondary role. And so there is a significant debate between Joseph's approach to the patient's history as useful in illustrating the transference now, and the classical approach which regards the transference as illuminating the past that is to be reconstructed now (Blass, 2011). Even the 'archaeological' explorations described in Chapter 9 only come from the close examination of the here-and-now process (or micro-process as Joseph saw it).

This view is not just a model of the psychoanalyst as a passive recipient, but as an active person seeking engagement. It is a demanding job that is required, and Melanie Klein referred to only half of it. She described (see Chapter 6) how she should learn about herself, but we also need to add that the learning must take place in a particular context – that context being the patient who has stumbled upon and activated some aspect of the analyst.

Hopefully, the analyst will have some clue as to what has been activated in himself, though he may find it difficult and requiring the silent work of self-analysis, as Money-Kyrle said (Chapter 5). Thus, we need to be aware that the role of the psychoanalyst's own analysis is not to prepare him for all eventualities, but to give him the grounding for continuing his analysis, even after his analysis has finished – 'post-graduate self-analysis', to use another of Money-Kyrle's useful phrases. The point of a training analysis is, therefore, not to do a complete analysis, which is impossible anyway, but to grant the analyst the ability to take it further on his own. The training analysis needs to instil a process, not simply the results. In other words, the analyst has to perform his 'double observation' method – observing what is going on in the relationship, and observe himself observing. Conducting a psychoanalysis is a reflective practice, but not what is usually meant by 'reflective' (Dewey, 1910). It requires a reflective speculation on the *unconscious* level as well as what is observed consciously. And so, countertransference is not eradicated in this view, it is material for the analyst's ongoing reflection (as in fact Melanie Klein conveyed to her younger colleagues – Chapter 6).

CHAPTER 11

The reflective analyst
What was that?

The analyst's job has expanded. It is no longer a matter of merely observing the speech and behaviour of the patient, and giving it a meaning. The analyst must now make a continuous observation of himself, making meaning of the patient's utterances and behaviour. As mentioned, the reflective practice here is a double observation. In this chapter, I shall emphasise especially the work of Irma Brenman Pick (1985) on what she called the 'working through' in the countertransference.

She explored extensively the disturbance the patient causes the analyst, and that the analytic work is not just powerful head-stuff in order to make meanings. It is work to make meanings *plus something*; plus work on one's own reactions – the 'silent piece of self-analysis'. She gave an example (pp, 158-160) of a man whose bitter defensiveness exemplifies the stultifying hatred he felt for the help he needed, infused in part by long experience of frustrations:

[He] had recently come to live in London, his first

analysis had taken place abroad. He arrived for his session a few hours after having been involved in a car accident, he himself just missed being severely injured. He was clearly still in a state of some shock, yet he did not speak of shock or fear. Instead he explained with excessive care what had taken place, and the correct steps taken by him before and after the collision.

Here is a picture of a defensive reaction that strangles the fear and shock. The moment had been deadened;

He went on to say that by chance his mother phoned soon after the accident, and... responded with 'I wouldn't have phoned if I'd known you'd have such awful news. I don't want to hear about it'.

The patient believed he had learned in his previous analysis to accept his mother's limitations:

He was, however, very angry with the other driver, and would pursue, if necessary to court, his conviction that [the other driver] would have to pay for the damage.

The patient conveyed very vividly how he bore his shock, fear and rage at the accident, and at his mother's reaction, carrying it on his own and remaining above it. The patient had done some learning, but as we noted, the analytic learning of his previous treatment had been to create this defensive competence, rather than a real understanding and insight into his rage at feeling neglected on a deeper level:

> Instead, he felt he had been taught to 'understand' the mother or listen to the analyst with an angry underlying conviction that the mother/analyst will not listen to his distress. He went along with this, pulled himself together, made a display of behaving correctly... bearing pain with competence in doing the right thing, but let us know that unconsciously he will pursue his grievances to the bitter end.

The analyst considered the process in detail.

> The patient made an impact in his 'competent' way of dealing with his feelings, yet he also conveyed a wish for there to be an analyst/mother who would take in his fear and his rage. I interpreted the yearning for someone who will not put down the phone, but instead will take in and understand what this unexpected impact feels like; this supposes the transference on to the analyst of a more understanding maternal figure. I believe though, that this 'mates' with some part of the analyst that may wish to 'mother' the patient in such a situation.

The analyst feels the ordinary maternal response of sympathy, but there is a complex situation. The analyst did want to give the maternal response which the patient longs for – should she comply (or not)?

> If we cannot take in and think about such a reaction
> in ourselves, we either act out by indulging the patient
> with actual mothering (this may be done in verbal or
> other sympathetic gestures) or we may become so
> frightened of doing this, that we freeze and do not
> reach the patient's wish to be mothered.

The countertransference, she shows, may lead us to be non-
analytic, or distancing, and these alternatives we have, need to
be thought about. One alternative seems to be a kindly, though
not insight-oriented, intervention; the other is remotely cool/
cold. They are quite understandable impulses; indeed what
could be more natural than an analyst who would like to ease
the upset in a motherly kind of way. But she said:

> I then needed to reflect about the parts of himself and
> his internal objects that did not want to know. These
> too were projected into the analyst, and also in my view,
> 'mated' with parts of the analyst that might not wish
> to know about human vulnerability (ultimately death)
> either in external reality, or currently in feeling 'tossed
> about' by the patient in the session.

The two alternatives – not wanting to know (or have insight),
or distancing and being competently above and beyond the
upset – may, she says, also be attitudes of the patient that she

joins in with, quite understandable ones. Either of the pair of alternatives could collude with some part of the patient that evaded his bitterness. The motherly analyst, on taking thought, could see that:

> [H]e believed that in presenting me with such an awful picture of mother/analyst, he persuaded me to believe that I was different from and better than them. Yet he also believed (and that was how he had behaved toward me at the beginning of the session) that I too did not want to know about the fear

This implies that:

> [W]e [can be], like the patient, in danger of 'wrapping it all up' competently... If we fail to take into account in statu nascendi our own conflictual responses, we risk enacting that which we would be interpreting, i.e. the hijacking of all the good propensities and the projection into the other 'driver' of all the evil; we may behave as though we could meet with accidents or the vicissitudes of life with impunity.

The role of being a competent interpreting analyst can work in nicely with the patient's competence, which he uses to assist the analyst emotionally, as well as himself. By simply interpreting, as is our job, we may be falling in with the required role of mutual competence as a defence.

Behind the projection, the analyst, if he takes thought, can make out problematic reactions the patient doesn't want to know about:

> In taking the case to court, the patient's belief in the superiority of competently keeping out passions and ostensibly pursuing 'pure' truth, needs to be examined. What looks like truth-seeking is suffused with [legalised] hatred. There is an underlying menace that if I make a wrong move, my name will be blackened, as he has already blackened the other driver, mother and the previous analyst.

I want to show in this how the analyst has to struggle with the deadening impact on the live experience of the patient and the live response of the analyst. That deadening, as Brenman Pick states, is suffused with a powerful litigious hatred kept out of view. It surfaces actually in the analyst's feelings of judging the mother and the previous analyst. The analyst has to keep alive this most natural response to the vulnerable patient's trauma and help the patient do so too – they both have to face the opportunity for litigious hatred. It is only by taking account of what one is impelled to 'do' that the analyst's side of the interpersonal clinical relationship can be worked through.

So, traveling in similar territory to Money-Kyrle's (1956), Irma Brenman Pick (1985) was describing the mobilization of the psychoanalyst's thinking as a kind of 'mating' between the two minds:

> If there is a mouth that seeks a breast as an inborn potential, there is, I believe, a psychological equivalent, i.e. a state of mind which seeks another state of mind (Brenman Pick, 1985, p. 157)

Thus, the patient seeks a *state of mind* in the analyst; and Brenman Pick exemplified this in the patient's seeking out a 'sympathetic' analyst who the analyst did in fact want to be – but could notice that she risked judging herself superior, 'a more understanding maternal figure... [that] "mates" with some part of the analyst that may wish to "mother" the patient in such a situation' (Brenman Pick, 1985, p. 159).

In this example, a reflective analyst works at being cognisant of the subtle pressures signified by her own wishes and feelings about the patient, and this entails being cognisant with her feelings about herself.

A silent piece of self-analysis

Money-Kyrle's (1956) comments about 'a silent piece of self-analysis', and Melanie Klein's (1958 [Spillius 2007]) view that countertransference 'helped me to understand myself better', chimed with Heimann's eventual (1960) warning about the wild use of the analyst's feelings.

The fundamental principle of psychoanalytic practice is that the analyst's reactions need to be dealt with in some way. We have moved on from the thick-skin, impassive blank-screen analyst and from the 1920s when the training analysis merely prepares the analyst to suppress his own reactions. This chapter has tried to illustrate how, from the 1950s onwards, the analyst has a way of making use of his own reactions – provided of course he works to understand them in terms of the material. The analyst's understanding of the material is indelibly shaped by an understanding of himself.

CHAPTER 12

And the reflective patient, also What does the patient see?

Implicit in the discussion in the last chapter is the fact that the object studied is at the same time a subject too. We are all psychologists; even the most disturbed of us. Whilst being a patient and displaying whatever he needs to be understood, he is just as alert to what the psychoanalyst is displaying, although he may feel he has less licence to engage in a discussion about his observations.

In Money-Kyrle's remarkably candid description of his case, he succumbed to an introjection from the patient, and remarked that as a result of his mistake, the process had moved on – 'a new situation arises in which his [the patient's] response to [the analyst's] mood may itself have to be interpreted' (Money-Kyrle, 1956, p. 363). Money-Kyrle represented the complex succinctly when the patient reacts to the countertransference, the analysis has to go on from there; he cannot go back to the *status quo ante* – 'it was useless to try to pick up the thread where I had first dropped it. A new situation had arisen which had affected us both' (Money-Kyrle, 1956, p. 363).

Money-Kyrle listed *three* things (Chapter 5):

- the transference,

- the psychoanalyst's reactive countertransference, and

- the patient's reaction to the analyst's countertransference.

This third element is not yet greatly explored (see Peräkylä 2010).

We have seen that if the analyst is on the track of the patient's unconscious phantasy, the chances are that, in his own way, the patient is tracking the analyst's thinking. The result is that whilst the analyst attempts to understand the patient's mind, so the patient at the same time is making his own observations and constructing his understanding of the analyst's mind, and then reacting accordingly. The patient will have his own receptiveness or lack of it.

However strong the analyst's commitment to the blank screen approach, the patient is still likely to find ample evidence of the analyst's personality, including the possibility of the analyst being hard-to reach. Indeed, the analyst's striving to achieve such a position will probably spark off expectations about the analyst's willingness to ride pillion on the patient's terrors and catastrophes. We should not under-estimate how well our patients get to know us – after all, they meet us every day over a period of years; we really cannot conceal much of our selves, however much we withhold actual facts.

Mistakes and cross-purposes

Debate occurs over the psychoanalyst's responsibility (or the patient's) for difficulties or lack of progress. It alternates between the patient's responsibility and his inherent 'badness', or alternatively the analyst's intrusive pathology. It may be a sterile debate as both patient and psychoanalyst are involved with each other in enacting the joint drama. This implies an equal engagement, almost a 'democracy', a two-way interaction, or 'mating' as Irma Brenman Pick called it. Whatever the resistance, it is with the unconscious collusion of the psychoanalyst. Some balance of responsibility seems most likely – and soothing to the analyst's professional super-ego. This moves us away from the pathologising of either, since both are complicit in the resulting dramas.

We will refer yet again to Money-Kyrle's (1956) case as a paradigm. There the analyst made interpretations that were not entirely convincing to him, he said – nor to his patient. Because the patient began to accuse the analyst, by the end he said, 'It was I who felt useless and bemused' (Money-Kyrle, 1956, p. 363). Any engagement between them to create understanding died. This result – only appreciated after the session – was the transfer of some feeling of uselessness from the patient who arrived with it and passed it (with his rejection and contempt) into the analyst who accepted it and went away with it. It was acknowledged that these problems occur 'whenever the patient corresponds too closely with some aspect of himself [the analyst] which he has not yet learnt to understand' (Money-Kyrle, 1956, p, 361).

The analyst clearly failed, understandably perhaps. The patient, on the other hand, was also complicit, communicating uselessness into the analyst, perhaps in the only way he could. In desperation, he found a place in the analyst to off-load a noxious experience. Some other mind was available or indeed was activated. Whatever the patient's motivation, for which he is responsible, it meets the analyst's responsibility for handling it.

However, if the analyst fails it is not just that he made a mistake – although he did make a mistake unconsciously. There is a situation in which the analyst accepts to be some evacuated part of the patient. As the patient said, 'this explained why he [the patient] had been so angry with me yesterday: he had felt that all my interpretations referred to my illness and not to his' (Money-Kyrle, 1956, p. 363). The patient actually recognised some part of the analyst at a moment when the analyst remained unconscious of it.

When the analyst gets caught up with the patient through these countertransference engagements so that joint enactments occur, the patient may be acutely aware of what is happening to the analyst. Three possibilities then arise: (a) the patient *incorrectly* sees his phantasies as truly happening to the analyst; (b) the patient *correctly* sees his phantasies matching the analyst's state of mind and behaviour; and (c) the patient is instrumental to some degree in '*creating*' the analyst's state of mind in conformity with his own phantasies. In any of these cases, from the patient's point of view, he is in relation to a mind that is in some respects disturbed. Enactments are thus a part of the patient's defensive system, and we are probably in the domain of Freud's transference cure.

Cross-purposes

The patient will seek evidence whether the analyst can face the suffering in question. That would require a powerful use of intuitive inspection into the analyst. The patient may succeed in spotting the analyst's ability, though of course his intuition may be faulty – no doubt it is at times. However, it is no doubt accurate at times, as the example of Money-Kyrle's patient was. When on form, the analyst creates a new situation for both, and does so with resources the patient has not found in himself – the analyst finds a new way to understand something unbearable brought by the patient, and puts it in words. Then the patient's sense of a helpful other bringing relief must spark off, not just gratitude and new-found moments of self-understanding, but also complicating experiences of jealousy and envy, vulnerability and defiance. In turn, the analyst will then be confronted by such a turmoil of responses that both please and dismay him – even when he only half understands them. On the other hand, when things 'go wrong', as they often do, the patient is confronted with an analyst who does not wish to be alive to the patient's distress.

Interpretations that, for the analyst, are insights generously offered are, for the patient, quite different. They may seem like openings into the working of the analyst's mind that tell the patient if he has done damage or not, and, maybe, give evidence to the patient of the analyst's resentment or retaliation – or forgiveness, or some other realised phantasy. It may be that the more disturbed the patient, the more acutely they scan the analyst's interpretations to assess what is happening to the analyst's mind.

Whilst the patient is formulating what he can find in the analyst, the analyst is using his unconscious phantasies to explore the patient. The constructions in the analyst's mind may not be as hidden as he thinks. It seems likely that we use different terms for the different parties. In other words, for the patient we speak of his unconscious phantasy, or the 'unthought known', or the unarticulated trauma; for the analyst, we might more grandly speak of his theories, including the analyst's barely conscious 'implicit theories' (as Sandler, 1983 called them; see also Tuckett et al., 2008).

As analysts, we are all floundering in the belief that our patients come for the insights we can offer. In fact, that belief so easily leads us into being at cross-purposes. The patient's unconscious seeks to buttress his defences, and the analyst seeks to understand them and what is behind them to defend against. Such cross-purposes are common enough (Hoffman, 1983; Aron, 1992; Greenberg, 1991; Gabbard, 1995; see also Rosenfeld, 1987; Schafer, 1997). Joseph warned that analysts must look 'at the way in which patients use us – analysts – to help them with anxiety' (Joseph, 1978, p. 223). These are active and subtle processes that ensure the analyst's consciousness is clouded, and that includes the peculiar quality of destructive hatred invested in the defensive reactions of many patients.

If the patient fundamentally believes that the distress is unmanageable by anyone, then they will expect, usually unconsciously, and with bitter resentment, that we will join them in their expectation of a collaborative evasion (Feldman, 1997). A patient needs his analyst to know about the suffering, and will engage in such a way that the analyst shall know clearly what the suffering feels like. At the same time, he believes the analyst will tolerate it no better than he has been able to. In fact, if the analyst can tolerate it, then the patient may feel the intolerability has not been sufficiently communicated. Fundamentally, the patient expects an analyst as defensive as himself (Hinshelwood, 1985), and will believe the analyst to be pretending and insincere if not as overwhelmed as the patient. He may feel his best option is to try to learn the analyst's methods of defence and evasion.

That the patient is dedicated to his own defences is understandable enough; he has found his pain and suffering to be beyond relief (the reason he comes to look for help) but cannot, of course, understand how anyone could do better with his pain than his own efforts. Patients may want an analysis, but only partly. Melanie Klein advised, 'we must understand what in the patient's mind analysis unconsciously stands for at any particular moment' (Klein, 1943, p. 637); and Joseph pointedly put it:

> After all, the reason which brings patients into analysis is fundamentally that they cannot manage anxiety (Joseph, 1978, p. 223).

At least, it takes time, and sometimes a long time, before the patient can gain some confidence that real help is at hand to achieve something he had believed impossible.

Since a psychoanalysis may not in fact stand, in the patient's mind, for what it does in the analyst's mind, it does not necessarily or consistently stand for self-understanding. We have seen that the very act of interpretation may be drawn into service in support of defences, even as we interpret them. Hoffman and Gill (1988) described such a case where:

> [T]he moment of interpretation itself is frequently invaded by the very features of transference-countertransference enactment to which the content

of the interpretation is addressed (Hoffman and Gill, 1988, p. 60).

So, the patient may be seeking non-analytic ends in his use of the analyst. Psychoanalysts use the term resistance – though I am speaking of one form of resistance – because they want to convey that there is an entirely reasonable sense in avoiding analytic understanding and in bitterly combating the wish for it, from the patient's point of view. A patient manages his anxiety as best he can. His method has failed in the past, and so his belief in his time-honoured means must remain undimmed, because he lacks alternative resources. He will inevitably use the analyst in accord with his past belief, however despairing. That defensiveness, and distortion of his objects, is, in fact, what we term transference, and is therefore what he will repeat. It does mean, however, that we have to be alert to his use of ourselves which opposes, or is tangential to, our expectation that the patient wants to gain insight.

I suggest he may even regard the pursuit of analysis as a reckless and dangerous path taken by the analyst, if unconsciously it means abandoning his past methods of coping. Often an initial part of the analysis has, therefore, to bring to consciousness the patient's belief that his experiences are indeed intolerable. The only sensible course for him then is to shore up his defences.

When the psychoanalyst does react to the patient with

disturbance, it may be completely understandable to both parties.

Deadening

A particular situation arises with many patients. They lull the analyst into thinking that he is conducting an analysis. However, it is too calm, seemingly too co-operative, but bland, and lacking in lively moments. In the end, it effects no change; the patient is not reached. The analyst may believe a great deal of work has been done, and indeed it has, but not analytic work. It is work that looks like the real thing, but it doesn't progress. Analysis starts only when it is realised that the analysis has not started.

This 35-year-old man had commenced analysis with quite a paranoid fear of being attacked. This had quickly taken the form of an anxiety in the analysis that my opinions put into his mind would obliterate his, and him:

> He started one session telling me he had not written a cheque for the bill I had given him the session before. He had come straight on to me this morning after a night shift he had started temporarily. He felt different today compared with when he came from home. After five minutes' silence, he then said a relative had told him a story about his mother passing a homeless man on the street and she refused to give money. He implied

this was very callous.

This view of his mother was familiar: someone who was distracted in her mind by other thoughts and problems she had.

I said it was a complicated situation. He was clearly distracted by his work from my need, expressed in my bill, but he then felt guilty about it, as if he was like his mother not giving to the homeless beggar in me. But I became aware that I was keen to interpret this link.

He responded in a slightly lofty way that he thought what a sumptuous area of London I live in. This may have been a simple denial, but I thought it carried something else. I wondered if my keenness to make the interpretive link felt to him as if I wanted to take over with my own lofty, superior thinking, so that he felt in danger of being obliterated. Perhaps I had indeed been a bit quick and realised that perhaps it was because I thought his announcement about the cheque had been a bit unapologetic.

As I was trying to capture this in my mind, he had gone on to another thought. He told me he had seen a beggar in the street on the way to me today. He said this factually as if he expected me to recognise a link with the earlier story of someone homeless. A moment later, he said it was more that he was worried about his own neediness.

I then made an interpretation based on an assumption that turned out to be incorrect. I assumed the conflict was about accepting an insight about neediness. So, I talked to him about the neediness in him, in the beggar, in me and in the people whom he looked after on the night shift. I was aware again of feeling some satisfaction with this interpretation.

He responded characteristically. He said being with me, was always like hitting a brick wall. I believed then that my assumption had been wrong. His conflict at that moment was not so much about insight into his neediness. Instead it was still his fight with an object in me, a mother with a brick-wall mind that ignored his, and was pleased with my own thoughts that I put into him.

I said he felt at that moment I was distracted by the importance of my own ideas, and, from what he had said, I reminded him of a mother who had no room to think about him.

Quite strikingly his moment of resentment vanished. He clearly felt remembered by this interpretation, and he then addressed his feelings of being under attack. It was not simply his neediness, but that when in need he was attacked by a mind that blotted him out.

It appeared there was the projection of a rich parent/mother into me, and my acceptance of this inflation that led me to protect it with a brick wall, he thought. He assessed my interpretation, my superior mind (and superior geography of my house), and believed that it was a brick-wall mind that needed to leave him out. This patient was acutely sensitive to whether the person he was with had a mind that was open to his distress. He saw a powerful anxiety in me too, that I had to protect my mind from his encroaching distress.

When my patient tried to use my mind as a place to put aspects of his own experience, he found that my mind refused to accept his experiences and his needs; and he then felt I turned the tables and demanded he accept the thoughts from my mind. This patient is occupied with an object that turns away from his needs and makes him feel guilty for burdening the mother in me, and also frightened of the retaliation. He had indeed assessed my mind correctly at that moment. In the end, I had given an interpretation of the patient's *analyst-centred* focus at the moment (Steiner, 1993). His changed response pointed to how much he needed his pre-occupations with my mind to be recognized. At the point I grasped this problem sufficiently for him to feel that his fears were in fact grasped, his manner changed and he discovered his own capacity to think about it. My verbal elaboration at that moment contained the immediate moment of distress about how my mind was functioning. As a result, he did regain his capacities for thinking, and for understanding himself for a while. The response to my interpretation did convey that it had been a valid interpretation, one that tallied emotionally with him at that moment. The moments I recorded demonstrate, I suggest, an interaction in which I did in fact have certain feelings of my own, to which I reacted. In this sense, I enacted with him an irritable intrusion into his mind.

The uniqueness of this approach is in the technical implications. It is a constant process by which the analyst is incorporated into the patient's phantasies of trying to reveal them. Of course, the patient does not only employ his/her reflective capacities for defensive purposes. Equally he requires and seeks true understanding; or he may feel driven to spare the analyst from his own turmoil; or indeed triumphantly deliver the analyst into just the very turmoil he suffers. What the precise motive for these particular manoeuvres of hard-to-reach people are, will be developed in the next chapter.

CHAPTER 13

Resisting the death instinct
What's the difference?

Freud's late and pessimistic paper on interminable treatments (Freud, 1937) considered the possibility of a deliberate resistance to giving up the benefits of treatment, and remaining stuck in the neurotic state. Though there are many possible reasons, this one, attributable to the essentially self-destructive working of the death instinct, is highly contentious. The particular motive, a *self*-destructiveness, takes the form of defeating the psychoanalysis – and the psychoanalyst. The result is either a failed analysis, or surprisingly often an enduring (but wasted) analysis that wallows in an impasse, as Freud observed.

The contentions about the death instinct lead to two general perspectives on these clinical situations;

- First is a view, like Freud's, that there is after all an implicit effect of the death instinct that becomes in fact clinically visible – i.e. the non-progress of the work; this has been especially promoted by Betty Joseph and those in her decades-long seminar (Hargreaves and

Varchevker, 2004).

- And the second view is that explored by Rosenfeld (1987), where impasse can be shown (at times at least) as a result of incorrect interpretation, and analyst incomprehension.

Reaching self-destructiveness

The difficulty that hard-to reach patients so frequently bring is that the patient brings his destructiveness to the analyst for help, but then presents it as the destruction of help. It is as if the analyst has to manage a double resistance, one that seeks to defeat him, and the other that insists on keeping at a distance any knowledge of that self-defeating and analysis-defeating process.

An instance of the first of these possibilities, the clinical entrance of the death instinct is in Joseph's (1975) seminal paper devoted to 'Patients who are hard to reach'. She gave an illustration (p. 78-79); this vignette started with her interpretation the previous day about the rather deadening and superficial atmosphere he seemed to create in the session. The interpretation had made him angry and upset, but he did later get some insight 'momentarily into his competitive controlling' (Joseph, 1975, p. 78). After his sense of having been helped, the next day he had a dream:

He dreamed that he and his wife were in a holiday cottage. They were about to leave and were packing things in the car but for some reason he was packing the car farther down the lane, as if he were too modest to bring it to the front door or the lane was too muddy and narrow. This was unclear. Then he was in a market getting food to take home, which was odd: Why should he take food if he were going home? He was choosing some carrots – either he could take Dutch ones which were twisted or some better French ones which were young and straight, possibly slightly more expensive. He chose the Dutch twisted ones and his wife queried why he did so.

This is a detailed dream and (without including the patient's associations here[8]) it gave an opportunity for an interpretation of the analyst's countertransference feelings of the lack of life in the session:

[The analyst] suggested that his pseudo-modesty about bringing the car to the door was really linked with the fact that he was not too keen that I should see what he packed inside, following the feeling of having been helped the day before. But now we could see that his attempts on the previous day to force me to interpret

8   This patient is discussed in more detail in *Clinical Klein* (Hinshelwood, 1994, p. 189-192).

in a particular way, as well as the understanding he had gained about it, had become linked with attempts to pack my interpretations inside himself, not to use for himself but for other purposes, as, for example, to use for a lecture which he was actually giving that evening. This then becomes food which he himself buys to take home, not food he gets from home-analysis. He chooses carrots which should help his night blindness, which should give him insight, but what he actually selects are the twisted ones. This would suggest that part of him has insight into his tendency to twist and misuse material — the false interpretations he tried to get from me – and avoid the clear, direct contact with firm, straight, fresh, and new carrots – that is, non-text-book interpretations. This insight is not yet felt but is projected into his wife, who queries why he has to do things in this wrong way.

There is, in this interpretation, the nub of the problem with this patient. He does listen to the interpretation the day before, even though painful for him. It is his unconscious that responds by producing a dream that gives some idea of how he manages to make the contact between himself and the analyst lifeless again. He takes the interpretation, but not with a gratitude or appreciation appropriate for something that tallies properly with his problems.

Instead, he can be seen to turn the analysis into something less than lively by choosing to twist the interpretation as he takes it in. He turned it (twisted it) into some intellectual idea to be exploited for quite different purposes other than insight into himself. He escapes the pain of self-knowledge and honest development, which might be the stuff of life. Instead, he steals and twists his analysis into something quite different from what the analyst thinks he comes for, and life is bled from the potential fruitfulness, leaving the deadness through which it feels hard to reach him.

The satisfaction in dealing with the pertinent interpretation in this way coincides with Freud's more speculative view of the negative therapeutic reaction – a more direct destructiveness towards the analytic help. In contrast, the possibility that the analysis gets stuck in another way is illustrated by Rosenfeld. Here, an incorrect interpretation is because the analyst does not understand the transference-countertransference situation. As we have seen in Chapter 12, the mistaken interpretation leads the patient to react to this occurrence in his own way – the analysis, as Money-Kyrle said, had moved on. Unless the psychoanalyst can realise his mistake *and* the way the patient has taken that mistake and reacted to it, there is a danger that the patient remains with a guilt-ridden construction of the analyst who sees the patient's construction as being a malicious misinterpretation (a twisting of the analyst). Rosenfeld (1987, pp. 140-141) illustrated this kind of enduring impasse with Eric, who after 8 years of analysis (prior to meeting Rosenfeld) had reacted with shock when the previous analyst had suggested they finish.

> Shortly after [the analyst's suggestion], he was suddenly overcome by strong feelings of contempt for the audience to whom he was at that moment lecturing. These feelings were so strong that he was scarcely able to finish the lecture… He was very shocked by the incident because lecturing had been an activity he always enjoyed…
>
> [This] experience at the lecture had an enormous impact on him and made him feel a very much increased need for help and understanding through his analysis. He… felt in a great dilemma because [the analyst] seemed to be as shocked and at a loss as he was about what had happened; and this may have been true… [H]e had not been able to detect any feeling of understanding in her. This impression may perhaps have been influenced by the fact that it appeared [the analyst] had concentrated her interpretations after the lecture incident almost entirely on the triumph and contempt, which she thought Eric, was expressing towards her. He reported for example,

that she said that he wanted enviously to destroy the success of the analysis and make her look entirely incompetent. Interpretations of this kind were felt by Eric as critical angry remarks which increased his hopelessness and isolation and made him feel unable to put anything in order.

In a way the analyst *was* critical – she was addressing a negative side of the patient. The analyst, in her own shock, could not retain the position of a listening analyst, and failed to take in properly what he was saying to her. She did not see Eric's reaction as disappointment, but as triumph. No doubt she was badly affected by failing with Eric and his unexpected catastrophic reaction, and like him she too could no longer conduct a learning situation. Interestingly, this static and torturing analysis continued 'over a number of years'.

Being anxious about the turn things had taken her interpretation may have lacked not just understanding of why it occurred, but a lack of understanding in the sense of not feeling *with* the patient. The outcome was to fulfil the interpretation of the negativity in the patient:

> [H]e had felt very critical of [the analyst] at the time. He felt she seemed to be unconcerned about the pain, depression, and hopelessness he was feeling. He wanted to have a second opinion… [However] he was

too frightened. He... felt threatened by her hostile power if he did not completely obey her.

Thus, an impasse developed over a number of years. The analyst then reduced the number of sessions to once a week, which Eric 'experienced as a further threat and as an illustration of [the analyst's] cruelty' (p. 141). So, Eric, had become increasingly sensitive to, and suspicious of, the analyst, and indeed interpreted her interpretations. Or rather, the patient *mis*interpreted her. He believed the analyst was not impelled by helpful intentions but by cruel and punitive wishes, delivered with words meant to hurt. Each had become a 'bad object' to the other.

Rosenfeld's careful reconstruction was aimed to show the emergence of this bad object relationship from the lack of understanding of the analyst, and the patient's reaction to the analyst's capacities and her reactions to him. These two clinical vignettes illustrate two sides of a controversy:

1. The wanton twisting of the insight for the purposes of a perverse (and deadly) destructiveness and

2. A mutual misperception in which the analyst failed to see the patient's true efforts so that the patient became defensive which the analyst misperceived as a triumphant and perverse destructiveness.

Defence as destruction

Another illustration attempts to see a different relation between defence and destruction, not an either/or dispute but a convergence into a phenomenon seen from two sides. This is Mr B, a psychologist, who was about 40.

> He was senior in his particular branch of his field, and with a good knowledge of psychoanalysis. He had had a previous psychoanalysis for 8 years, and came to me because he felt that he often lacked the feelings he should have, and that they must be inaccessibly bottled up.

> He was always frank with me about himself, and gave no impression of concealing or resisting. For instance, he was quite willing to talk of a possible homosexual interest in a friend he had once worked with. He could talk as intelligently and with as much psychoanalytic sophistication about himself, as I could. He was clearly impressed by his own ability to be frank, and in a lofty way would tell me such shameful things with a superiority which presumably compensated for any shame. He was not boring, in fact, his words revealed quite a creative way of expressing himself, and his interest in himself was contagious.

But he experienced himself as emotionally blocked. And so did I. When a family tragedy occurred to relatives, he knew it was a tragedy. In the ensuing rituals he played his part efficiently, but he did not know if he really felt how affected he was. He had no tears. In fact, he had not had tears since he was a child.

He started a session, the first one after a break over Christmas, not long after he started with me, by talking about his father-in-law who had rung up one day very anxious and distressed because his elderly wife had collapsed. The father-in-law was very troubled because the doctor had not arrived, and he felt abandoned with this crisis and did not know what to do. My patient went on to talk of a colleague who had left the country. That man had left his wife and children when he emigrated, but was due to return for a brief period to see the children. However, he missed the flight. My patient thought that the children would be distressed.

He was telling me of the abandoned feeling that both his father-in-law and his friend's children felt. Commonly, after a break in analysis, patients talk of distressed and abandoned people, who usually represent the patient's feelings, which have been denied. When that is interpreted, either a patient will become thoughtful and appreciate something new in himself, or he will resist the interpretation strongly. However, it was not so with my patient.

He simply agreed that their distress may represent his about the break. The problem with his agreement was that it seemed merely on the surface. My interpretation did nothing to put him in touch with any live distress. Indeed, it seemed as if those abandoned people he talked about were not *representations* of something in him at all. In other words, his distress was no longer in him. It was in *them*, and gave him an opportunity to display his superior articulateness.

> At this point, faced with his bland agreement, I decided to point out the difficulty of locating his distress. He agreed with this too, in the same unruffled way. He talked then of something being locked up in him – he talked of a sealed 'box' inside him. His appreciation of the problem was sophisticated, and he understood the unusual structure of his own mind. Curiously, I found myself engaged and interested in this division in his personality and how clearly he was describing it. I was responding to a strong move on his part to establish securely a professional self – a self that that can discuss *about* himself.

I was in a curious state. On the one hand, I felt my interest aroused by the problem that his case posed, and about which he could talk eloquently. At the same time, I felt a strong frustration. This man managed his distress by requiring everyone else around him to experience it, except for himself. As a psychologist, he knew enough intellectually to interest me. But, as a personality, he could unconsciously use me to support his psychological sophistication with creative discussions. I thus assisted his habitual method of avoiding any depth of emotional knowledge of his experiences – and he endured a largely shallow or deadened experience of life and of himself.

We can question the persistence of the 'shallow' professional discussion in place of insight, and whether this was, on one hand, a perverse self-destructiveness that wantonly turned (twisted) the insight into intellectual fodder to make it useless but impressive, or if, on the other hand, it was a tired but highly necessary defence against seeing too far into his anxieties and conflicts.

The patient produced emotional-sounding material. The analyst gave what he thought the patient was in need of – interpretations. Both parties danced together whilst preserving a distance from a vivid engagement. They were not meeting. He eventually told me a dream I took to be significant:

> In the dream, he was in a house with some people. A Dr X was examining a wall and recommending that

a hole or doorway is made in the wall. Through the hole a view would then be seen. That view would be a spit with meat cooking on it, there was some rusty old machinery which might be useful as a barbecue. Further away across a country valley were some houses, a village. But all the houses were leaning over. He realised that his own house was leaning too.

He described Dr X as a practical person, a problem-solver. Also he knows Dr X's wife in real life as well. She is a busy person who is always feeding people.

Later he recalled that he knew Dr X's wife is a work colleague of mine.

The relevance of this dream to my theme is twofold. Firstly, it is clear that he has some thoughts about breaking out of his 'sealed box' – the hole in his wall. The dream does convey that, unconsciously, he has some awareness of what he needs. He needs to see a feeding situation – though that is pictured as a denigrated rusty old bit of machinery. There are here two components, the box defence, and the denigrating reduction of the feeding apparatus.

In a second thought coming immediately after the need to feed – the result of Dr X's, or my, efforts to expand the patient's view – was a destabilisation of the world – it leaned over precariously. It is as if to view his own neediness would be extremely destabilising, and generates the defensive need to wall off any view of that neediness. This is a stark warning from the patient of imminent collapse – and is he wrong?

He is appealing, unconsciously, for help to avoid a calamity – perhaps a fear of insanity – definitely a defensive motivation. So, one use of the analyst would be the support of his brick wall. By finding in me a willingness to discuss interpretations with the sophisticated psychologist in him, I am the kind of support that protects his psychic box – his professional identity – against the calamity.

At the same time, there is a connected theme. The apparatus that provides the needed sustenance is rusty and old, and thus denigrated. And it occurred to me quite convincingly at times that his confidence in his rather superior manner of expressing himself left me in a role of a rather rusty old analyst who, maybe, was held at a distance being out of my depth with such a gifted patient. His pride in himself at his knowledgeable fluency did two things: (i) it kept a box-like brick wall defence against real insight, and (ii) this prideful view of himself had the impact of a destructive demolition of me.

The point of this clinical story is the way *both* defence and destruction occur in the one process of mobilising the analyst in this way. They are bound up together, a defence against the destabilising 'seeing', *and* the destructive denigration. Both motives – frustration and self-defeat – coincided in one dream, in one psychodynamic process. In other words, we may not have to separate the defence and the destructiveness as two aspects in opposition.

Resistance and destructiveness

Resistance, defensiveness and death instinct aggression seem to go together in these patients in a coherent way. This is open to dispute. And no doubt my clinical illustration is open to alternative understandings. So, a brief word can be added on the debate over frustration versus destruction. Some analysts who are averse to the idea of inherent innate destructiveness may choose to emphasise understandable defensiveness; others committed to envy and other manifestations of death instinct will emphasise the destructiveness and self-destructiveness. However, it may be more moderate to accept that they combine together. So, a satisfaction in undermining arises from two sources simultaneously in these patients, both, (i) defending against the intolerable, and (ii) mobilising a satisfaction in destructiveness.

Thus, defences may be driven by an innate destructiveness, just as satisfactions are driven by innate love and desire. There is no reason why love should be allowed its status as natural, whilst destructiveness is not, yet many psychoanalysts from different schools will dispute the provocative term 'death instinct'. In contrast, the life instinct is much more acceptable. When a mother feeds her little baby we are quite willing to accept that the feelings of satisfaction, appreciation, contentment and coherence, a sense of wholeness, arise from the life instinct This is not balanced with the opposite view, if mother does not feed at the moment of need, then there is a different reaction in the little baby, so that screaming intensifies, frustration and rage escalate, the arms wave frantically in uncoordinated ways, the baby leaks its tears with abandon. That equal and opposite instinct, a deadly one, is more difficult to accept in the baby. Each reaction seems no less innate and pre-formed at birth than the other. A similar descriptor to the innate 'life instinct' could make *semantic* sense; the opposite term, 'death instinct' would seem quite appropriate. Both are just as visible from the start.

However, many would dispute this simple symmetrical terminology, and claim an innateness about the first – the life instinct – and baulk at the innateness of the diametrically opposite – a death instinct. That view would have it that the reaction is 'frustration' of the life instinct – which it undoubtedly is. However, in coldly logical terms, the idea that frustration brings out 'death instinct' is no more far-fetched than the idea that satisfaction brings out the life instinct. It is unlikely that there would be much dispute about the different occurrences. The observation of the baby's opposing states of mind and feeling, and their occurrence from the very beginning of life, seems incontrovertible. There is no real reason why agreement over the observations should lead to disagreement over terms. Disagreement must come from other sources. A kind of squeamishness exists – perhaps understandably – when considering determined destructiveness in the earliest emotions of the sweetest baby.

Part 3 Conclusions

The chapters in Part 3 have tried to demonstrate the vulnerability of the psychoanalyst, as a person, to becoming embroiled in the interactive dynamics of the patient's unconscious (as well as his own). The patient is confined to a role in this same unconscious processing as well.

Although some schools of psychoanalysis referred to previously as within the co-constructivist trend try to redress perceived power imbalances, these efforts are almost always at a conscious level. In fact, the power in a psychoanalysis – in the work of the analysis – is with the patient's unconscious. However, the analyst is not entirely dependent on the guidance of the patient's unconscious. The account here of the usefulness of the countertransference points to the way an analyst may be aided in understanding his own communicating unconscious. To do so, he might consider any deadening experience, a deadening of what might seem like potentially live moments.

At that point, a loss of enlivenment, the analyst might bear in mind that he and his patient have, for the moment, formed a 'fit' (or mating) between transference and countertransference. This could set the analyst thinking that he has reached a point where it will be worth considering the countertransference. He might suspect he is involved in a role that will demonstrate a narrative significant for the patient. He should consider those dead or stuck moments as an inevitable enactment.

The unconscious speaks unconsciously. Moreover, it is heard unconsciously. And the countertransference appears to be one of the most important decoders of those coded communications, and lies beside other methods of decoding, such as Freud's method of analysing dreams.

The use of countertransference is essentially a form of process analysis, and displays a narrative with (at least) two roles. This playing out of a narrative has a lot in common with the narratives played out with toys in a child analysis. It contrasts with the thematic analysis of dreams, and of free associations. This conclusion introduces the final part of this book, which emphasises the necessary importance of process, and the role of 'countertransference', outside of the clinical context. Working with hard-to-reach patients has provided a magnifying glass for examining the process aspect of the work as it is going on; it is a sort of bottom-up approach, as opposed to a theory-driven top-down approach.

PART 4

REACHING BEYOND

So far, the emphasis has been on how the psychoanalyst enters his work every day, *as a person*, vulnerable to being moved, and also relatively resilient to those pressures. In Part 4, we will look in the opposite direction. If the countertransference plays such a part in the unconscious process in a session, to what extent can our learning be applied outside of the sessions, back into ordinary life?

So, these chapters will discuss the way that the clinical notion of countertransference has been taken seriously beyond the therapeutic aim. First of all, the view that countertransference represents an especially intimate connection between persons, in which each can unwittingly play roles for each other, leads to rather radical questions about the nature of individuality and of personal authority, and ultimately of ethical practice in a psychoanalytic treatment (Chapter 14).

Then in Chapter 15, we consider the role of countertransference in defining and collecting research data. Following Heimann's view, that countertransference can be checked against the actual material in the session, we have the possibility of making use of triangulation, two perspectives converging on a unique occurrence in the analytic process. This characteristic – that countertransference and free association material can be used as checks against each other – enables precise pinpointing of narrative aspects of the session that may be used as reliable data for rigorous research (Hinshelwood, 2013a). In fact, as we will see, countertransference can both inform and check interpretations, so that as an element of triangulation, it functions as a refinement of interpretations in clinical work itself as well as in research results.

When working with psychoanalytic ideas (such as countertransference) in several different settings beyond the psychoanalytic clinic, we must recognise the limitations of our concepts. It was always Freud's dream that psychoanalysis would push way beyond the clinic and become the basic human and developmental psychology, as well as the standard philosophy of mind and aesthetics. He got into trouble with his claims for the psychoanalysis of everything. His followers tend, for various reasons, mostly in our unconscious, to over-claim through an idealisation of psychoanalysis. After all, we have put our all into it. The reality is that we should reign ourselves in; we, psychoanalysts, can contribute in many realms on the basis that there is an unconscious element to many issues, problems and conflicts; we can contribute to them, and no-one else can. However, that unconscious realm is *all* we can contribute.

Nevertheless, in areas such as group therapy, and the dynamics of organisations that conduct stressful tasks, intractable problems occur, apparently without solution from conscious thought; then it is worth considering whether investigation of the unconscious level needs attention. Then psychoanalysis is the essential resource for tackling those mysterious moments when unconscious processes surface so often unhelpfully and psychoanalytic thinking is the only discipline that can help at that hidden level (Hinshelwood 2001b, Hinshelwood and Skogstaf 2000,).

CHAPTER 14

Morals and ethics
Who has the authority?

The discovery of countertransference in the clinical setting prompts the question whether such intimate and powerful unconscious pressures occur outside the work of clinical psychoanalysis. And if so, what do they look like? This chapter reviews some of the evidence for the occurrence of countertransference-like unconscious processes in ordinary life and their implications for ethical and political behaviour.

The fluid structure of a personality

From his attempts to understand group dynamics, Freud was aware of the fluidity of the self, the structure and identity of the ego. He started his book (*Group Psychology and the Analysis of the Ego* 1921) with the work of Gustav LeBon, a French social psychologist. Freud quoted him:

> The most striking peculiarity presented by a psychological group is the following. Whoever be the individuals that compose it, however like or unlike be their mode of life, their occupations, their character,

or their intelligence, the fact that they have been transformed into a group puts them in possession of a sort of collective mind which makes them feel, think, and act in a manner quite different from that in which each individual of them would feel, think, and act were he in a state of isolation (LeBon, 1895, quoted in Freud, 1921, p. 72-73).

It is clear from this that Freud thought his understanding of the unconscious could explain how its pressures push group members into playing specific roles which they might not take up elsewhere, just as the psychoanalyst may be pushed into playing a role for a patient.

This phenomenon can be found in quite ordinary people in quite ordinary situations, and when it does, we hardly recognise them. Freud saw this kind of personality change in the state of a hypnotic trance:

[T]he ego becomes more and more unassuming and modest, and the object more and more sublime and precious, until at last it gets possession of the entire self-love of the ego. . . . The object has, so to speak, consumed the ego (Freud, 1921, p. 113).

That is to say the ego, or self, gives up its functions for reflection, self-assessment and self-determination:

> [T]he criticism exercised by that agency [the ego-ideal]
> is silent; everything that the object asks for is right and
> blameless. . . . The whole situation can be summarized in
> a formula: *The object has been put in the place of the ego ideal.*
> [The personality] is impoverished, it has surrendered
> itself to the object. (Freud, 1921, p. 113).

Here the ego-ideal is silenced as if it is missing and lost, and
the person depleted. But more, Freud saw the passionate state
of being in love as a parallel example of this depletion.

> From being in love to hypnosis is evidently a short
> step. . . . There is the same humble subjection, the same
> compliance, the same absence of criticism, towards
> the hypnotist as towards the loved object. There is the
> same sapping of the subject's own initiative (Freud,
> 1921, p. 114).

The depletion, loss of initiative, loss of judgement, and the
surrender to the other person exemplify the way the ego,
even in ordinary circumstances, may vary its functions at the
unconscious level – producing palpable changes in experience,
behaviour and autonomy.

This implies a serious breech in the integrity of the personality.
Personal authority cannot be relied upon. Quite normally,
when I go to work, I accept the authority of my boss, he has

authority, and that means he can make work decisions for me. My own self-determination goes out of action in a temporary way. In addition, those who are subordinate to me will accept my decisions about the work we do. This fluidity of changes in ego functioning appears to be normal enough; so normal, in fact, that we don't think about it. The ego takes up very different positions, and may change swiftly from moment to moment, when, for instance, I go from my boss to my assistant.

One way of looking at this is in terms of primitive mechanisms. Just as those mechanisms redistribute roles within the psychoanalytic setting, so, in social life the primitive mechanisms split up the person. Then, parts may be located elsewhere in others who perform functions for the subject.

The fragile coherence of the self

Now, from a psychoanalytic point of view, what is going on when the ego, or self, shows such virtuosity in adapting to different degrees of autonomy and paternalism? When we think of the personality structure, comprising id, ego and super-ego, we assume a fair degree of stability. We do not usually think of the ego itself as being manoeuvred into various social forms. Yet that is the conclusion to be drawn from the points Freud was making, and indeed from these general observations any of us can make (Hinshelwood 1997c).

It is not that the ego merely solves conflicts that occur between the other agencies of the mind – the id, the super-ego, and reality. Instead, we seem to have strong evidence that the person (his ego) is fundamentally destructured in itself from time to time. This is a different level of unconscious dynamics – beneath the Oedipal level of unconscious conflict, there is a deeper level concerned with the very coherence of the self. The subject under hypnosis literally *loses* his active self.

Silvia Amati writes of extremes, the dictatorships in South America where the torturer in such regimes aims at an extreme disturbance of personal integrity; he:

> … seeks to provoke breaches in the identity, i.e., in the sense of internal cohesion and continuity. . . . [T]he torturer's aim is to destroy thought and identity (Amati, 1987, 112).

The Stockholm syndrome (Ochberg, 1978), as it is now called, is an example of the extreme depletion of judgement and abject surrender.

These effects can be most effectively explained with the concepts of primitive mechanisms, just as countertransference appears to be the manifestation of those mechanisms in the psychoanalytic clinic. The primitive mechanisms split the ego and parts may be evacuated, or projected out, and then seen in others.

Freud was aware of a fluidity of the structure of the ego, for instance in 1927 he described a 'splitting of the ego'. He illustrated this from his understanding of the psychic nature of the fetishist who splits his ego. In this case, the ego can deal with the fear of castration by splitting into two parts, each part employing different defences; one defence denies the apparent 'reality' of female castration, and the other defence accepts it. Clearly to accept and also to deny requires a double vision, and Freud thought that the ego of the fetishist exists in two parts that were incapable of coming together. This is not a *conflict* over whether women are castrated or not – a straightforward conflict implies that the points of view come together, and clash. The situation Freud described was where there was *no* conflict, no coming together, but an aloof neglect of the other split part of the ego.

In the 1930s, others followed this up, speculating on the coherence of the ego. Edward Glover (1935) thought that the ego started as separate nuclei (each nucleus forming around the separate organs of perception). Then, in the course of development, they come together in a coherent structure. Donald Winnicott (1945) also thought that the initial ego was unintegrated. Melanie Klein (1946) considered Winnicott's view and decided it was wrong; the initial ego is coherent and whole, but becomes disintegrated and split subsequently as part of the very earliest defences of the new ego.

Of course, no one can know the earliest ego at this depth, and the debate is so speculative it is worthless to continue. But in later life, such as that of the adult fetishist, there appears to be a secondary process that actively splits up the ego – rather than a regression. Klein postulated this process of active splitting (as opposed to just falling apart) on clinical evidence, especially from adult psychoanalyses she reported in 1946. She associated the 'splitting of the ego' with, on one hand a splitting of the object, and on the other the primitive defences of projection and identification.

Beyond countertransference

This versatile inconsistency of the ego has consequences of various kinds. Not only is the role of the psychoanalyst compromised, but roles in ordinary daily life are as well. Transfer of parts of the ego from one person to another is commonplace. An example that is fairly easy to identify with is the following:

> A teenage girl, for example, who says "Dad, I'm going to stay out till two o'clock tomorrow morning. And I'm going to that disco, the one which was busted for drugs", and then waits, apparently innocently unaware, for Dad to say something. Her announcement is likely to have made Dad rather anxious. Dad, having his daughter's best interest at heart, will dutifully get

worried and tend to admonish and advise good sense about getting home early, about what company to keep, and so on. The teenager, although perfectly capable of assessing the risks for herself, has blissfully shed this, for the time being. Instead of feeling anxious, she has engaged with a specific part of her father which allows her to split off and lose a capacity for mature judgement. She can project it into her father because she knows he will introject the worry and will respond in a certain worried way; this is the responsible and protective father in him. It is not that she is unable to judge the risks involved. On the contrary, it is because she 'knows' the risks in her plan for the evening, that she needs her father to worry about them, rather than suffer the worry herself.

This is an everyday example, at least for a family. The transfer by projection and introjection complicates the exercise of authority and indeed the very acquisition of adult autonomy and authority are compromised.

At the opposite extreme, there are unconscious roles that are taken up in psychiatry, with a redistribution of responsibility. This is also familiar enough. Psychotic mental health problems show the same kind of loss, but on a much more dramatic scale. Here is an example: A psychiatrist admitted a patient who had caused worry about herself with her outrageous behaviour.

> She had been continuously stripping off her clothes; she had spoken repeatedly of life-saving, of her interest in magnetism, that her mother was dying (which she was not), and that her son would become a priest and "be able to help". As if this was not sufficiently unintelligible to the admitting doctor, the circumstances preceding her admission were also not immediately clear, since she had collected a black-eye from someone (not her son) in the process of becoming ill and arriving at the hospital.

> The feelings induced in the doctor and nurses were of the woman's wildness and unpredictability and that they were called upon to manage her, to control her and, above all, to stop the incessant flow of unintelligible chatter. In common parlance, they felt called upon to *'shut her up'*... we may note that whatever the anxieties and opinions of those outside the hospital, these had now to find resolution within the hospital... the patient does not suffer her pain, rather as intolerable anxiety, of being bereft of self-control, it is projected into the hospital staff who are engaged to suffer it for her. The staff then deal with it... as best they are able, generally altogether ignorant as to the sources of the patient's

anxiety – indeed, they scarcely even recognise it as anxiety (Conran, 1985, p. 36).

The patient, when so full of highly exciting disturbance, had lost control of herself. Her own control had gone missing. Instead, the staff and the hospital came to have control of her. There is a transfer of autonomy. Staff suffer the alarm of the patient's disturbed experience; they must embody what the patient has lost. This patient had lost her self-care function dramatically, and in an intrusive manner so that staff had to perform that control for her.

In terms of the primitive mechanisms, the patient had *split* her ego so that her capacity for making good judgements was *projected*, or evacuated. Her behaviour was so alarming and dangerous that it forced others to take care of her. Others were compelled very powerfully to *introject* the function of keeping her safe. Clearly, the staff were forced to take over a kind of parental function, and performed her own function of self-control for her.

Social and interpersonal consequences of ego incoherence

With such distortions of ego function, how does one decide when a person is sufficiently able to make a decision – even for himself – and when is he not? A debate has endured over several generations about the age at which new adults should be given the vote, and the example of the adolescent above gives an indication why this is more complicated than on the surface.

Psychoanalysis is radical for its insistence on the unconscious levels that determine thought and behaviour. Even issues of power are seriously hampered by such complications. Are the psychiatric staff the powerful ones with the force of the law and the Mental Health Act behind them? Or is she, the patient, the powerful one because she has forced the others to act in the way they did? Power can no longer be discussed in general terms, we must specify in any debate what sort of power is being considered.

The patient we have just considered was not an autonomous person, in the sense that she could not be relied on to make good decisions and to be responsible for herself. She lacked *her* own authority, and thus the functions that are involved in looking after herself. That function had been lost, and yet, not quite. It did continue, but in the minds of other people. The confusion of self, of who was looking after her, makes the issue of responsibility and autonomy complicated. This has ethical implications in psychiatry (Hinshelwood, 2015); what level of ego depletion would one regard as compatible with functioning as a responsible citizen, and what level would require some sort of custody? With extreme cases like the woman just described the decision is not so hard to make, but where is the boundary? The adolescent is in no way suffering a psychotic disorder, but may still not be a fully responsible citizen, at least in some respects. So what respects count for what purposes? – a complicated case-by-case discussion is required, it would seem.

For a long time, troubling social psychology experiments have followed up those kinds of changes that LeBon observed – influences such as those that emerged in the work of Solomon Asch (1952) on group opinions versus solitary dissenters; and of Stanley Milgram (1963) on coerced obedience. They showed how group pressure could induce irrational and alarming behaviour in a member of a group. These influences and pressures from social forces are not trivial. Serious, and expensive, public opinion makers set out to create a voting public who are compliant to certain views (alarmingly, it is the views held by those who have the money to pay opinion formers).

The rhetoric on democracy assumes, erroneously, that most persons are satisfactorily autonomous in their political thinking and voting. But it is not so; in fact, we all come under considerable outside pressure that is applied with the quite conscious aim of subverting personal authority and independence of thought. Manipulative influences are used in the public media, and sometimes the social media, and this has a long history. Edward Bernays, one of the founders of the public relations industry, (and, incidentally, Freud's nephew) wrote a book on propaganda in 1928. One quote from it seems sufficient:

> The conscious and intelligent manipulation of the organized habits and opinions of the masses is an important element in democratic society. Those who manipulate this unseen mechanism of society constitute an invisible government which is the true ruling power of our country (Bernays, 1928, p.10).

He was referring to the public relations industry in his country at the time (the United States). That industry is the 'invisible government' of a democratic society.

This brings us back to the role of countertransference. Whereas we have discussed how patient and analyst can get into an impasse as they operate at cross-purposes, there are ethical issues in this. If the patient prefers to live on with strengthened defences rather than to work through psychoanalytically revealed insights, then it might be regarded as unethical to continue working with him. Or to put it another way, if the patient consciously wants to learn about psychoanalysis, but unconsciously wants to avoid insight, then which part of the personality do we take our cue from, the conscious or unconscious? Indeed, even a patient who has given a pretty much informed consent will, we know, resist as well, and will show an informed *dissent* at certain times. Ethically, we might debate our position at these times, and whether we should simply carry on carrying on, or whether there are issues to consider in the decision to continue (Hinshelwood, 1997c, 2014).

Patients in the psychiatric service

Mental healthcare workers are particularly disconcerted by the work they do, and they are not neutral at all (Gordon and Kirtchuk, 2008; Hinshelwood 1999b, 2004). A 'contagion' occurs:

> Nurses are confronted with the threat and the reality of suffering and death as few lay people are... [But the] objective situation confronting the nurse bears a striking resemblance to the phantasy situations that exist in every individual in the deepest and most primitive levels of the mind (Menzies, 1959, p. 46).

A care organisation develops a particular culture of care practice – staff and inmates (Miller and Gwynne, 1972). Here is a general description of such a professional culture:

> ... only roles of health or illness are on offer; staff to be only healthy, knowledgeable, kind, powerful and

active, and patients to be only ill, suffering, ignorant, passive, obedient and grateful. In most hospitals staff are there because they seek to care for others less able than themselves, while the patients hope to find others *more* able than themselves. The helpful and the helpless meet and put pressures on each other to act not only in realistic, but also fantastic collusion... [The] helpful will unconsciously *require* others to be helpless while the helpless will *require* others to be helpful. Staff and patients are thus inevitably to some extent creatures of each other (Main, 1975, p. 61).

These inter-related group roles evolve unconsciously, and deliver care based on depersonalised roles. Take for instance the following occurrence:

The patient was led into a quiet room for her relaxation therapy. She remained there with her nurse, who locked the door, and pressed a button on a tape machine which played for 20 minutes. The nurse sat down and appeared bored from over-familiarity with the tape. At the end the nurse, wordlessly, switched off the machine, unlocked the door and led the patient out.

The role of care was interpreted as merely semi-custodial; keeping the door locked, switching on the machine. Any personal quality to this care functioning was pre-empted by the strictly mechanical interpretation, and exemplifying the quality Erikson called 'distantiation'. In a remarkable book by Hardcastle et al. (2007), the interpersonal distancing is revealed in conflicting unselfconscious accounts by both users and carers:

> When I first arrived on the hospital ward two male staff took me to a side room. I desperately wanted to go to sleep. I hadn't slept well for two months... One was clearly more senior than the other and he wrote in the book whilst the other went through my belongings... After this job had been done, the junior one (who later told me he was a bank nurse, 'What's a bank nurse?') stayed in the side room with me. 'Why?' He started chatting about his personal difficulties. He may have thought this would be helpful....
>
> I wanted to sleep
>
> .... He continued to talk. I was worried that if I told him to stop he wouldn't like me (Hardcastle et al., 2007, p. 23-240)

As Brenman Pick (1985) cautioned, the analyst moved by his own feelings risks becoming either frozen in rejection (as the nurse in charge of relaxation therapy), or compelled to be human (illustrated in the next vignette).

A team of carers involved in the rehabilitation of a serial offender released from prison (Davies, 1996) was drawn into quite unconscious role-playing. The team became blind to what happened to them:

> A disturbed man, Bill X, had a harsh mother as a child. She was violent and humiliated him. When released from prison where he had finished a sentence for brutal sexual crimes, he asked to be kept inside. The request was naturally refused. He subsequently engaged with the helping network in a specific way.

> He was dangerous and a specific plan had been set out at the hostel he was to go to, to ensure that only male staff dealt with him. However, the arrangements quickly broke done for extraneous reasons. He was taken into intensive counselling by a female worker; and a female prison visitor, who had visited him in prison, continued to see him, including taking him to her home where he assaulted her. Another female worker offered counselling, sometimes in evening sessions, and afterwards said she had forgotten he was a rapist! The female staff had been drawn into taking up powerful professional roles with him, to be inviting, and then to withdraw into professional work, giving him an intolerable feeling of powerlessness again.

So, the care network responded disastrously to his continuing disturbance. The staff did not seem to realise that the arrangements had broken down.

What went wrong could be traced very specifically to a repetition of the experience of care the man had as a child. His mother was very powerful and controlling and continually made him feel powerless; he had effectively no father with whom to identify. His sense of male power was unpractised and uncontrolled. In the hostel the male staff had disappeared – changed job, or went on courses, comparable to the ineffective father – and the female staff did their best to take over, as mother had.

The staff seemed unable any longer to think about the client realistically, or even to remember his case fully. The fairly simple professional insight that his violent and humiliating criminal activity is connected with treatment he received from his mother seems never to have been usable.

The staff did not realise how they had forgotten the prediction of the man's potential violence, and the initial caution of the staff. The man's demand was treated with a 'care' response, but not a reflective one. It was a sentimentalised sympathy, which passed as maternal caring, but in the event became his experience of maternal humiliation. It resembles the discussion by Irma Brenman Pick (Chapter 11) about the analyst who also found herself moved towards being a sympathetic mother rather than a professional analyst. Unless some thought can be sustained, the team must succumb to inappropriate professional identities, playing out roles for the client unconsciously. But in this case they had abandoned professional thinking in favour of a 'human' (or sentimental) caring. Thus, the work of the team and of a whole service can be said to be affected by a comparable process to that in a psychoanalysis.

This is a 'countertransference' on a collusive scale. The culture of psychiatric services has increasingly adopted an objective view of patients. This has features suggesting a defensive reaction to the stress of mental healthcare, and the unfortunate, and unthought consequences (Hinshelwood, 1999b). Scientific explanations of disease processes are substituted for the incomprehension the patient arouses. The depersonalisation of scientific psychiatry unhappily matches the inherent existential loss of self, characteristic of psychosis, and a self-defeating fit can enhance the long-lasting chronicity of the condition.

Another comparable example of a cultural 'fit' between a disturbed condition and the psychiatric service is that of severe or borderline personality disorders (SPD). As Malcolm Pines wrote:

> [We feel] impelled to conform to a pattern imposed by the patient, so that we begin to feel provoked, hostile, persecuted and [have] to behave exactly as the patients need us to, becoming rejecting and hostile (Pines, 1978, p. 115).

The angry rejection by the carer often confirms the life experience of such patients whose carers have in fact proved rejecting, abusing or worse. Characteristically, these patients have a personal history of childhood abuse from the people who are supposed to care. Unsurprisingly, they mis-identify carers as abusers, and both parties end up reacting in role (Norton and Hinshelwood, 1996, p. 723).

Thus, professional carers – not merely psychoanalysts, but psychiatrists and mental health nurses – may also be subjected to powerful unconscious forms of relating demanded by their charges.

Power in psychoanalysis

Since Foucault, there has been a lot of suspicion that psychoanalysis is a set of clinical power relations that assert the dominance of the professional in a coercive way. This power picture can be compared with the psychoanalyst's frequent sense of his weakness and uncertainty when on the job. It is also apparent from the discussions of countertransference in the clinical work, how much the analyst himself is just as much 'coerced' powerfully by unconscious processes into roles beyond his professional one.

Perhaps only a psychoanalyst can know the analyst's own sense of helplessness whilst waiting for signs of a patient's unconscious co-operation, a dream, say, a slip of some kind, a clash of contiguous associations, and so on. And indeed because we too are only human there may be an impatient hurrying on to something more active and powerful to dispel the experience.

In other words, the power in a psychoanalysis – in the work of analysis – is with the patient's unconscious. The psychoanalyst cannot work without its co-operation, and guidance. Much of course could be made of the question, who decides when the patient's unconscious is speaking, and what it is saying. This is not an idle question. There are patients who seem to have a particular attitude to insight. As John Steiner wrote:

> I want to make a distinction between *understanding* and *being understood*, and point out that the patient who is not interested in acquiring understanding – that is understanding about himself – may yet have a pressing need to be understood by the analyst. Sometimes this is consciously experienced as a wish to be understood, and sometimes it is unconsciously communicated. A

few patients appear to hate the whole idea of being understood and try to disavow it and get rid of all meaningful contact. Even this kind of patient, however, needs the analyst to register what is happening and to have his situation and predicament recognized (Steiner, 1993, p. 132).

In these patients, the capacity for insight can be said to have been split off and relocated *in* the analyst, without interest in any return of the lost curiosity and responsibility. The act of interpreting then solidifies the analyst in the role of the one who is interested in insight – a passion that drives the analyst. The patient has little trouble off-loading his own curiosity into that curious part of the analyst, which is on show with every interpretation.

CHAPTER 15

Research data

How 'true' is countertransference?

Freud thought research was crucial:

> In psycho-analysis there has existed from the very first an inseparable bond between cure and research. Knowledge brought therapeutic success (Freud, 1926, p. 256).

On the whole, psychoanalysts have followed in this direction, seeking new knowledge that is to be the engine of continuing success. This chapter will consider how countertransference has become an important instrument for collecting research data. With the recognition now of the role of countertransference as the experimental 'probe' of investigation, in conjunction with Heimann's warning to check the countertransference against the actual material, it is potentially possible to use the analyst's personality as the observing instrument. I argue that the psychoanalyst's personality is the receiving apparatus of data, albeit subjective data, that can supply research evidence (Hinshelwood, 2013a).

What research?

In recent years, psychoanalysts have been caught somewhat unawares by the demands on us by health providers and insurance companies for outcome research. Freud's five major cases do not comprise a sample of successful outcomes. Dora was a failure; Little Hans was hardly a 'treatment', just conversations aimed at conceptual research; the Rat Man did improve, a success. In the Schreber case, Freud (1911) analysed a book; and the Wolf Man remained in analysis most of his life with a string of analysts after Freud. Freud was not trying to show the effectiveness of psychoanalysis; Freud was after new knowledge.

New knowledge delivers greater success, and he meant that new knowledge must be put in the possession of the patient for him to succeed in his treatment. The patient's knowledge must be of his unconscious, and Freud embarked on the creation of psychoanalysis by introducing patients to this hidden area of themselves. He called it insight, of course. It was always possible for psychoanalytic treatment then to be reduced down to applying theories to patients – or fitting patients to Freudian theory. In fact, Freud did operate somewhat in this way. In this he, and psychoanalysis, proceeded rather in the traditional mode of German psychiatry, which, medicine-like, sought to place patients into categories, a diagnostic form of psychiatry.

Perhaps it is not surprising that he did tend to conform to the assumptions of his cultural context.

The Dora case early on began a hesitancy about this, because she showed the importance of *process* in the clinical work. Because of something going on between him and Dora, the patient ended up moving along a certain path (in Dora's case, she left treatment). Without being entirely sure of what he meant, Freud followed up that experience much later with an idea about working through, a process necessary for using insight, and not just having knowledge. Only at the very end of the paper does he give some idea of what working through is, in general terms, by comparing it with hypnosis.

> This working-through of the resistances may in practice turn out to be an arduous task for the subject of the analysis and a trial of patience for the analyst. Nevertheless, it is a part of the work which effects the greatest changes in the patient and which distinguishes analytic treatment from any kind of treatment by suggestion. From a theoretical point of view one may correlate it with the 'abreacting' of the quotas of affect strangulated by repression – an abreaction without which hypnotic treatment remained ineffective (Freud, 1914, 155-156).

Psychoanalytic knowledge is sterile unless it is brought into some active and alive process. However, at this time (1915, though not published until 1917) he wrote his paper on 'Mourning and melancholia'. There he described more explicitly the bit-by-bit withdrawal of the cathexis of, or involvement with, the lost loved one (the withdrawn libido to be directed eventually towards another object). The object-presentation (as he calls it – in effect the inner representation) is:

> made up of innumerable single impressions (or unconscious traces of them), and this withdrawal of libido is not a process that can be accomplished in a moment, but must certainly, as in mourning, be one in which progress is long-drawn-out and gradual. Whether it begins simultaneously at several points or follows some sort of fixed sequence is not easy to decide; in analyses it often becomes evident that first one and then another memory is activated, and that the laments which always sound the same and are wearisome in their monotony nevertheless take their rise each time in some different unconscious source. If the object does not possess this great significance for the ego – a significance reinforced by a thousand links – then, too, its loss will not be of a kind to cause either mourning or melancholia. This characteristic of detaching the libido bit by bit is therefore to be ascribed alike to mourning and to melancholia; it is probably

supported by the same economic situation and serves the same purposes in both (Freud, 1917 p. 256).

This is process thinking in fact, even though it is put in the contrasting terms of the economic model, terms such as 'cathexis'. It describes the systematic de-coupling of 'a thousand links' and letting go by a bereaved person. It contrasts with categorisation as the antithesis of process. I would argue that only when the recognition of the importance of the object as something interacted with, could process thinking develop and move away from simply fitting patients to theories. It has been the impact of taking a relational concept such as countertransference seriously that has allowed the attention to process to flourish further.

In one sense, this debate between categorisation and process thinking has become irrelevant, because, increasingly, factors in the wider culture of healthcare prioritise outcome. Certainly outcome is a process, but unfortunately it involves a process of changing categories, moving patients from an unhealthy category to a healthy one. It is different from the dynamic process that Freud attended to in his description of mourning a lost object.

Outcome or research and development (R&D)

In fact, the emphasis on outcome is a mirage. In the

pharmaceutical industry, where the insistence on outcome arose, there is another equally important research component – the research and development (R&D) as it is called, which produces the products whose outcome then has to be assessed. The research and development in psychoanalysis is the knowledge generated in the clinic. In psychoanalysis, R&D is just as important as the test of effectiveness. Drug companies and psychoanalysis need R&D, and we need to be familiar with how our own brand of R&D works. It doesn't have to be a method copied from science or anywhere else:

> Different disciplines have their own methodologies, procedures for systematization, while sharing overall, basic aims such as precision, completeness, representativeness, sharp contrasts (*Kontratschärfe*), transparency of observation and hypothesis testing (Leuzinger-Bohleber and Target, 2002: 3-4).

We have a good method for developing new knowledge – our clinical method. Clinical work is where our knowledge came from in the first place. Unless we stand by that clinical method of research, we will end up with nothing to work with clinically. But developing new knowledge is not a problem in psychoanalysis, it is apparently not difficult. Even from the early days of Freud's Wednesday meetings, there were new theories pressing on the group, notably Adler's, and later those of Bleuler and Jung at the Burgholzli Hospital.

Then, Freud performed the evaluative function of judging one theory against another. He did so on the basis of his own personal authority, but today, quite rightly, the authority of the expert is no longer appropriate (Hacking, 1999). So, psychoanalysis needs a formal method of critical discrimination – the authority of evidence, as opposed to the authority of experts. In any case, there is no one of Freud's stature to perform the function personally by sifting through the mosaic of theories that now constitute psychoanalysis.

After the early disappointment with Jung, Freud's authoritarian grip controlled what would, or would not, pass as valid psychoanalytic theory. Whilst certain incipient divergences did appear in different geographical centres, after he died the current plethora of competing psychoanalytic theories, often at war with each other, mushroomed. As Tuckett saw, years ago:

> After seventy-five years it is time not only to review our methodology for assessing our truths, but also to develop approaches that will make it possible to be open to new ideas while also being able to evaluate their usefulness by reasoned argument. The alternative is the Tower of Babel (Tuckett, 1994a. p. 865).

The need is for comparative work (Hinshelwood, 2010, 2013a). Do we need a figure of authority again, as Freud was? It is not likely to happen. So, how do we do it, now?

A paradigm for comparative testing

The market leader in research design is natural science. It is often said that psychoanalysis cannot hope to adopt that kind of model. For a start, we have only single cases to study, and cannot amass a significant sample with control subjects as well. Then the intimacy of the study is so subjective that it is believed no good data can be collected for research purposes. Although these criticisms are rather generally accepted, it is not without challenge (Ezriel, 1956; Edelson 1984, Hinshelwood, 2013a).

In fact, in a paper celebrating the centenary of Freud's birth, Henry Ezriel described the carefully controlled clinical process in psychoanalysis as logically identical with the experimental process in a natural science laboratory. Ezriel's long-forgotten claim deserves to be remembered. He described the process of a psychoanalytic session as proceeding from before an interpretation to after it. That process, he argued, more or less exactly fits the similar controlled process of a laboratory experiment in natural science, the initial laboratory conditions are set up; an intervention is made; and a change ensues. In the analytic process, the intervention is the interpretation. A brief example is familiar – when Anna O had her hysterical symptoms, Breuer intervened with a session of hypnosis. The symptom invariably disappeared or changed. This was so dramatically like a scientific experiment in general medicine that it impressed Breuer, and inspired Freud.

So, a change following the psychoanalytic interpretation indicates the validity of that intervention. The response to the interpretation can be assessed according to a set of 'operational rules'. Today, we no longer intervene with hypnosis. Our interventions, and interpretations, are based on analytic theories. Therefore, the clinical 'experiment' not only indicates the validity of the interpretation, but it infers a validity for the theory on which the interpretation is based. Ezriel gave a simple example:

> One of my patients started a session by unconsciously giving vent to hostile feelings towards me in the form of an attack upon the Government. After my interpretation he criticised the Clinic. The object of his attack had thus moved nearer my consulting room, from Whitehall to the Tavistock Clinic (Ezriel, 1951: 33).

Ezriel's operational rules specified that a *required relationship* (in which, in this case, the focus of an attack is distant, in order to prevent an *avoided relationship* (an immediate attack upon the present analyst), because the avoided attack might lead to a *catastrophe* – the analyst may succumb to the attack. If the interpretation was correct (and the theory behind the interpretation – in this case, Oedipal rivalry), then after the interpretation, the narrative will move explicitly towards the here-and-now relationship with the analyst. In fact, such a process can give results with a single experiment in natural science. Likewise, a psychoanalytic theory can be shown to be effective with only one case.

Countertransference as subjective data

However, Ezriel left it to intuition to compare the initial, required relationship with the subsequent avoided relationship, and thus to assess the change. Today, we are in a position to make this comparison much more precisely than an intuitive stab in the dark. Using the double perspective of (i) countertransference process plus (ii) the narrative in the content of free association, a precise assessment of the before and after is possible.

There is an important caveat about comparing the preceding and subsequent narratives. The crucial test is the *change in the common narrative* (of process and content) before interpretation, compared with after. Pre- and post-interpretive narratives should be the same – so that in the example, the narrative about a fatal outcome of an Oedipal conflict is common before and after the intervention (interpretation). The change after the interpretation is that the patient can better assess the reality of the narrative that was initially so impelling for him.

Where there is a change in the overt and conscious narratives of the two modes, then that is not a positive result. It is a change from some other influence, a false positive. It is not possible to claim that *any* change can be happily reported as a positive result. The change must be in line with a specific prediction based on the narrative of the preceding material. Otherwise, a change will be a false positive. Indeed, no response to interpretation claimed in the literature to be significant should be simply accepted until that change in the underlying common narrative has been demonstrated (see Hinshelwood 2013a).

The data from this triangulated method is not immune from error, and subjective wish-fulfilment, but it is probably as immune as most natural science observations. If this is granted, then we have a method for testing the validity of theories. This is R&D, the generation of our grounding theories to be used in clinical work.

The subjective receiving apparatus

I gave an example in Chapter 3 of a middle-aged man, who told me of a meeting with an unreliable friend. The interpretation was incorrect, but the illustration continued and shows how the correct interpretation, when it was given, could be shown to be correct. Here I repeat the section already given in that previous chapter:

> He told me of a meeting he had with a friend with whom he was working on a project. The friend did very little towards the project, rarely contributed what he had agreed to do, and was in fact a very unreliable man. However, my patient was extraordinarily fond of and loyal to this friend. On this occasion I found my-self thinking what an unreliable patient I had, who at times would literally go to sleep on the project I was conducting with him. I felt a mixture of irritation that I was struggling so much to make headway with his analysis. I interpreted this a little mechanically along these lines. I compared how we both struggled to keep a project going, him with his friend, and I with him. He was silent (in fact a common response for him), and then he started snoring (also common).

I had seen my irritation at struggling with the analysis (the countertransference), and his project with the unreliable colleague (the actual material) as the single common narrative, and interpreted how we both struggled to keep a project going. The subsequent response to the interpretation was that he was silent and then started snoring.

I took this as a failed interpretation. Had the interpretation been correct I would have predicted an unconscious change in the struggle in the analysis, both less irritation in my countertransference, and actual material that suggested more co-operation. That prediction clearly did not happen. Then, continuing, when he woke:

> He remembered what he had been talking about, and the interpretation. And he courteously acknowledged the link I had made. I felt he was reassuring me, even patronising me a little. He continued to tell me how he had worked with his friend all evening and well into the night, whilst, interestingly, the friend had gone off to bed. He explained how the friend needed a lot of encouragement and reassurance, and his own role was to be very tolerant whilst he did most of the work.

Whilst I was thinking about his reassuring me, he continued to tell me how his friend needed so much reassurance and encouragement. Then I could see another double story. First in the countertransference, I felt I was being encouraged, and second I heard the same story of encouraging his friend, in his actual material. So continuing with my notes:

> Then I interpreted that he was trying to tell me that he felt he had to be very tolerant of my limited abilities to contribute to the analysis in the way he had expected and needed. Yet I said he felt very loyal me and he had

to keep things going.

The question now is what was his response to that? In fact, it was quite different.

> This time he did not go to sleep. He changed the subject and said, he had been very interested in two insects flying in the room where he had been working, and he had been trying to estimate the difference in the buzz of each which gave him some thoughts about the project he was working on – it was a musical project. I was heartened by his change of topic as it made me think that something was moving on.

What I saw here was a significant change, and a change in line with the prediction. The prediction was that the narrative of a lack of co-operation would move towards a more co-operative narrative. There was indeed material about co-operation – the two insects buzzing around together. And in the countertransference? – well, I felt more heartened. I both felt a more co-operative and hopeful feeling, and I listened to the story of the buzz between two 'busy bees'.

I present this as a triangulation – the content and countertransference indicated a narrative evolving from less to more co-operation. I take this to be a positive experimental result, not because he changed the subject, but because the change was specifically in line with the move to co-operation, which was predicted on the basis of the narrative of the initial material. I can argue on the basis of this example that it is possible to check subjective observations. This very abbreviated account of a psychoanalytic research design is a summary of a book length account, *Research on the Couch* (Hinshelwood 2013a)

Conclusion

Given that the field of study in psychoanalysis is a subjective one, dealing with the interactions between two subjectivities, it is fairly obvious that the instrument for observation should be a subjective one. Subjective data was termed 'immaterial facts' by Caper (1988). Generally speaking, subjective data is not measurable, they don't stretch through the three dimensions of space, and their location cannot be pinpointed by measurements. However, there are qualitative differences — and qualitative difference is often much more distinctive than quantitative ones. The presence or absence of one of Anna O's symptoms is more distinctive than something that may measure 1½ centimetres or 1¾.

So, a central feature of our methodology is the subjective instrument, that is, our selves. We make dual observations — first, the associations we listen to, and second ourselves as we do our listening. It is the latter that is subjective, and it means that countertransference is the true core of a subjective scientific method. This method indicates a proper check on the subjective experiencing of the analyst as the instrument for gathering research data. This is not research into outcome effectiveness, but it is basic research, R&D. In psychoanalytic research, the knowledge to be tested by outcome studies is that gained in clinical work, as Freud claimed in the quote at the beginning of this chapter. Clinical research in the treatment setting has always been the R&D of psychoanalysis.

CHAPTER 16

Conclusion
Now about the question...

This book started with questions about the experiences of alive moments and dead ones in the psychoanalytic process; Do they exist? What do they mean? What to do about them?

I recall as a young psychoanalyst, qualified in 1976, that I first encountered Bion in a lecture he gave at the Institute of Psychoanalysis in 1979, when he was on one of his regular visits to London from his sojourn in Los Angeles. The lecture opened with the rather dramatic description of the moment of first meeting at each session. It must be seen as a wildly turbulent event, 'When two personalities meet an emotional storm is created' (Bion, 2014 [1979], p. 136). This is extreme of course, but it called attention to the powerful impact minds make upon each other. He said this of course to jolt the psychoanalyst from a complacent, and mechanical process, too reminiscent of the doctor (or 'physician' as Bion would call him) or the scientist, who, by relegating emotional subjectivity from their supposed objectivity, is more like a psychotic than is supposed. Perhaps I've never quite lost the impact of that challenging statement, and how his turmoil knowingly contrasted with the assumed professionalism of my teachers (analysts and supervisors as well).

Many people have found it difficult getting over the impact of Bion's ideas. For me, the challenge was that patients and analysts are not so different, and perhaps I was sensitised by my decade or two of working in therapeutic communities where the interest is focused on the joint and socially shaped struggles that staff and patients make together in a communal way.

Much later of course, I realised that Bion's first supervisor during his own training was Paula Heimann, who did more than most in rehabilitating countertransference. I have wondered in my mind if his position was uncomfortable with a loyalty to his analyst Melanie Klein, whilst he must have felt at home with some of Heimann's central teaching. The emerging quarrel at the time between Klein and Heimann must have been an intensely personal introduction for him to the inter-tribal warfare of the British Society, not so distant from his own experiences of warfare. It was probably not a live moment that Bion felt was easily manageable, and led at first to his immersion in an epistemology of psychoanalysis (from about

1959 to 1965), and eventually his recourse to an advanced reliance on his own subjectivity as the best approximation to the unknown (the 'O'), or invariant of humanity.

Perhaps the single most important point from the discussion of this whole book is Freud's tally argument. The accent must be that interpretations should tally with something *in the patient* – not something in the analyst. The work in a psychoanalysis is, as Bion says, a storm for both parties. Clearly, as the psychoanalyst's mind is stormed, he/she inevitably needs to make sense of what happens in this close encounter. Intimacy requires work to 'survive'. To his relief, the analyst has many resources for performing this survival work. However, the metapsychological theories are a major element of those resources and so, the serious temptation is to concentrate on whether the theories can make sense of the material. It appears at times that less emphasis is placed on whether the understanding is actually relevant for that patient at that moment.

So tempting is the resort to the calming use of theories that developing new theories can seem to take on a priority, with the (thankful) neglect of the storm. It is not surprising that the prevailing modes of discourse, and the pressures for objectivity, prioritise the more sophisticated formulations of theory.

The crucial point is that the analyst's subjectivity is a powerful instrument for two opposing things (Britton and Steiner 1994) –

1. A motivation for making sense of the experience, the relationship, the process, and

2. Also a very potent source for jumping to conclusions, a force for ignoring whether the meaning is really the one that makes sense for the patient.

And we need to follow the, now well-emphasised, advice to *check* the countertransference. It is important to select as strictly as possible the truth of the countertransference as seen via the patient's unconscious.

Not only is there a divisive jumping to conclusions about metapsychological theories, but there is a similar dispute about the nature of countertransference itself. Whether we follow an intra-psychic intersubjective view of the analytic relationship or the co-constructivist view, the need is to privilege the patient's unconscious, not the patient's conscious, experience rather than the analyst's experience (conscious or unconscious).

The irony is that the zealous campaigning that psychoanalysts do on behalf of one side or other of these disputes is probably wasted steam, since in most instances (perhaps every instance), the position needs a more dialectical framing. Both Melanie Klein and Paula Heimann were probably right.

Countertransference is a tool, a probe, for investigating and testing, but it is a flawed instrument from which one can learn as much about oneself as about the other. We need to approach the intra-psychic versus co-constructivist positions as if there is an enriching dialectical structure to be evolved.

References

Aguayo, J. and Malin, B. 2013) *The Los Angeles Seminars*. London: Karnac.

Almond, R. (2003) The Holding Function of Theory. *Journal of the American Psychoanalytic Association*, 51:131-153,

Amati, Sylvia (1987) Some thoughts on torture. *Free Associations 8*: 94-114.

Aron, L. (1992) Interpretation as expression of the analyst's subjectivity. *Psychoanalytic Dialogues* 2: 475-507.

Asch, Solomon (1952) *Social Psychology*. New Jersey: Prentice-Hall.

Atwood, G and Stolorow, R. (1984) *Structures of Subjectivity*. Hillsdale, N.J.: The Analytic Press.

Austin, J.L. (1962) *How to Do Things with Words*. Oxford: Oxford University Press.

Balint, A. (1936) Handhabung der Übertragung auf Grund der Ferenczischen Versuche' *Internazionale. Zeitschrift. fur. Psychoanalyse 22*: 47-58.

Balint, M. (1950). Changing therapeutical aims and techniques in psycho-analysis. *International Journal of Psycho-Analysis*

31: 117-124.

Bálint, A. and Bálint, M. (1939). On transference and counter-transference. *International Journal of Psycho-Analysis* 20: 223-230.

Baranger M, Baranger W. (1983) Process and non-process in analytic work. *International Journal of Psychoanalysis 64*: 1-15

Barrett, R. (1996) *The Psychiatric Team and the Social Definition of Schizophrenia.* Cambridge: Cambridge University Press.

Bernays, E. (1928) *Propaganda.* New York Liveeright.

Benedek, T. (1953) Dynamics of the countertransference: *Bulletin of the Menninger Clinic 17*: 201-208.

Bentinck, A (2015) *Karl Abraham: Life and Work, a Biography.* London: Karnac.

Berger, P. and Luckman, T (1966) *The Social Construction of Reality.* London: Penguin.

Bion, W.R. (1954). Notes on the Theory of Schizophrenia. *International Journal of Psycho-Analysis* 35: 113-118.

Bion, W.R. (1957) Differentiation of the psychotic form the non-psychotic parts of the ego. *International Journal of Psychoanalysis 38:* 266-275. And republished in Bion

(1967) *Second Thoughts*. London: Heinemann.

Bion, W.R. (1959). Attacks on Linking. *International Journal of Psycho-Analysis 40*: 308-315.

Bion, W.R. (1962a) The psycho-analytic study of thinking. *International Journal of Psycho-Analysis* 43:306-310.

Bion, W.R. (1962b) *Learning from Experience*. London: Tavistock.

Bion, W.R. (1965) *Transformations*. London: Heinemann,

Bion, W. R. (2000 [1979]) Making the best of a Bad Job. In Bion, F. (Ed) *Clinical Seminars and Other Works*. London: Karnac Books.

Blum, H. (2007) Little Hans: A centennial review and reconsideration. *Journal of the American Psychoanalysis Association 55*: 749-765.

Blass, R.B. (2011) On the immediacy of unconscious truth: Understanding Betty Joseph's 'here and now' through comparison with alternative views of it outside of and within Kleinian thinking. *International Journal of Psycho-Analysis* 92: 1137-1157.

Bollas, C. (1989) *Shadow of the Object: Psychoanalysis of the Unthought Known*. London: Free Associations (and New York: Columbia Univ. Press.

Brabant, E., Falzeder, E. and Giampieri-Deutsch, P. (1993) *The Correspondence of Sigmund Freud and Sándor Ferenczi, Volume 1* (1908-1914). Cambridge, MA : Harvard University Press.

Brandschaft, B., Doctors, S. and Sorter, D. (2010) *Toward an Emancipatory Psychoanalysis: Brandschaft's Intersubjective Vision.* London: Routledge.

Brenman Pick, I. (1985) Working through in the counter-transference. *International Journal of Psycho-Analysis 66*: 157-166. Republished in Elizabeth Spillius (ed) (1988) *Melanie Klein Today: Volume 2, Mainly Practice*: 34-47. London: Tavistock.

Britton, R. and Steiner, J. (1994) Interpretation: Selected fact or overvalued idea? *International Journal of Psycho-Analysis 75*: 1069-1078.

Brown, J.F. (1936) *Psychology and the Social Order.* New York: McGraw-Hill.

Busch. F. (2015) Our vital Profession. *International Journal of Psycho-Analysis* 96:553-568.

Busch, F. and Schmidt-Hellerau, C. (2004) How can we know what we need to know? Reflections on clinical judgment formation. *Journal of the American Psychoanalytic Association* 52: 689-707.

Caper, R. (1988) *Immaterial Facts*. New York: Jason Aronson.

Carotenuto, A. (1984) *A Secret Symmetry: Sabina Spielrein between Jung and Freud*. New York: Pantheon.

Carpy, D. V. (1989) Tolerating the countertransference: a mutative process. *International Journal of Psycho-Analysis* 70: 287-294.

Casement, P.atrick (1985) *On Learning from the Patient*. London: Tavistock.

Cavell, M. (1998a) In response to Owen Renik's 'The analyst's subjectivity and the analyst's objectivity'. *International Journal of Psycho-Analysis 79*: 1195-1202.

Cavell, M. (1998b) Triangulation, one's own mind and objectivity. *International Journal of Psycho-Analysis 79*: 449-467.

Cavell, M. (1999) Response to Owen Renik. *International Journal of Psycho-Analysis 80*: 1014-1016.

Civitarese, G. (2008) *The Intimate Room: Theory and Technique in the Analytic Field*. London: Routledge.

Coltart, N. (1986). 'Slouching towards Bethlehem' or thinking the unthinkable in psychoanalysis. In *The British School of Psychoanalysis: The Independent Tradition*, ed. G. Kohon. New Haven, CT: Yale Univ. Press, pp. 185-199.

Conci, M. (2010) *Sullivan Revisited – Life and Work*. Trento: Tangram.

Conran, M. (1985) The patient in hospital. *Psychoanalytic Psychotherapy 1*:31-43.

Cushman, P. (1994). Confronting Sullivan's Spider – *Hermeneutics and the Politics of Therapy. Contemporary Psychoanalysis 30*: 800-844.

Davies, R. (1996) The interdisciplinary network and the internal world of the offender. In Christopher Cordess and Murray Cox (Eds.) *Forensic Psychotherapy, Volume 2*. London: Jessica Kingsley.

Dewey, J. (1910) *How we think. Boston: D. C. Heath and Company.*

Dunn, J. (1995) Intersubjectivity in psychoanalysis: A critical review. *International Journal of Psycho-Analysis 76*: 723-738.

Dupont, Judith (1988) Ferenczi's 'Madness'. *Contemporary Psychoanalysis 24*: 250-261.

Edelson, Marshall (1984) *Hypothesis and Evidence in Psychoanalysis.* Chicago: Chicago University Press.

Eizirik, C.L. (2010) Analytic practice: Convergences and divergences. *International Journal of Psycho-Analysis 91*:371-375.

Erikson, E.H. (1950) *Childhood and Society.* New York: Norton.

Erikson, E.H. (1956) The problem of ego Identity. *Journal of the American Psychoanalytic Association 4*: 56-121.

Etchegoyen, R.H. (1988) The analysis of Little Hans and the theory of sexuality. *International Review of Psycho-Analysis 15*: 37-43.

Ezriel, Henry (1951) The scientific testing of psycho-analytic findings and theory: the psycho-analytic session as an experimental situation. *British Journal of Medical Psychology 24*: 30–34.

Ezriel, Henry (1956) Experimentation within the psychoanalytic session. *British Journal for the Philosophy of Science 7*: 29-48.

Feldman, M. (1997). Projective Identification: The Analyst's Involvement. *International Journal of Psycho-Analysis 78*:227-241

Feldman, Michael (2009) *Doubt, Conviction and the Analytic Process.* London: Routledge.

Feldman, Michael and Spillius, Elizabeth (1989) Introduction to Part 2. In Joseph, B. *Psychic Equilibrium and Psychic Change.* London: Routledge.

Fenichel, Otto (1941) On transference and counter-transference. *Psychoanalytic Quarterly 10*: 682-683.

Ferenczi, Sandor (1988) *The Clinical Diary of Sandor Ferenczi.* Cambridge, Mass: Harvard University Press.

Ferro, A. (1999) *The Bi-Personal Field.* London: Routledge.

Ferro, A. (2005) *Seeds of Illness, Seeds of Recovery.* London: Routledge.

Freud, S. (1894) Obsessions and phobias. *The Standard Edition of the Complete Psychological Works of Sigmund Freud, Volume 3*: 69-82. London: Hogarth.

Freud, S. (1953 [1891]) *On Aphasia.* London: Imago.

Freud, S. (1905) *Fragments of an Analysis of a Case of Hysteria. The Standard Edition of the Complete Psychological works of Sigmund Freud,* Volume 7: 1–122.

Freud, Sigmund, (1909) *Notes upon a Case of Obsessional Neurosis. The Standard Edition of the Complete Psychological works of Sigmund Freud, Volume 10*: 153-249. London: Hogarth.

Freud, Sigmund, (1911) *Psycho-Analytic Notes on an Autobiographical Account of a Case of Paranoia (Dementia Paranoides). The Standard Edition of the Complete Psychological works of Sigmund Freud, Volume 12*: 3-82. London: Hogarth.

Freud, S. (1912) Recommendations to physicians practising psycho-analysis. *The Standard Edition of the Complete Psychological Works of Sigmund Freud, Volume 12*: 109-120. London: Hogarth.

Freud, S. (1914) Remembering, repeating and working through. *The Standard Edition of the Complete Psychological Works of Sigmund Freud, Volume 12*: 145-156. London: Hogarth.

Freud, S. (1915) The unconscious. *The Standard Edition of the Complete Psychological Works of Sigmund Freud, Volume 14*: 159-215. London: Hogarth.

Freud, Sigmund, (1917a) *Mourning and Melancholia. The Standard Edition of the Complete Psychological works of Sigmund Freud, Volume* 14, 239-258. London: Hogarth.

Freud, S. (1917b) Lecture 28, Analytic Therapy, *Introductory Lectures on Psycho-Analysis. 1916-1917. The Standard Edition of the Complete Psychological works of Sigmund Freud, Volume* 16: 448-463. London: Hogarth.

Freud, Sigmund, (1918) *From the History of an Infantile Neurosis. The Standard Edition of the Complete Psychological works of Sigmund Freud, Volume 17*: 3-122. London: Hogarth.

Freud, Sigmund (1921) *Group Psychology and the Analysis of the Ego. The Standard Edition of the Complete Psychological works of Sigmund Freud, Volume 18*: 67-143. London: Hogarth.

Freud, S. (1926) The question of lay analysis. *The Standard Edition of the Complete Psychological Works of Sigmund Freud, Volume 22*: 177-258. London: Hogarth.

Freud, Sigmund (1927). Fetishism. *The Standard Edition of the Complete Psychological Works of Sigmund Freud, Volume 21*: 147-158. *London: Hogarth.*

Freud, S. (1937) *Analysis Terminable and Interminable. The Standard Edition of the Complete Psychological Works of Sigmund Freud, Volume 23*: 209-254. London: Hogarth.

Fromm, E. (1970) *The Crisis of Psychoanalysis*. Chicago: Holt, Rinehart, Winston.

Foucault, M. (1980) *Power/Knowledge*. Brighton: Harvester Press.

Gabbard, G.O. (1996) The analyst's contribution to the erotic transference. *Contemporary Psychoanalysis* 32: 249-273.

Gabbard, G.O. (1995) Countertransference: The emerging common ground. *International Journal of Psycho-Analysis* 76: 475-485.

Gabbard, G.O. (1997). A reconsideration of objectivity in the analys.. *International Journal of Psycho-Analysis* 78: 15-26.

Ginsburg, S.A. (1991). The Clinical Diary of Sándor Ferenczi. *Psychoanalytic Quarterly* 60: 292-296.

Gitelson, Maxwell (1952) The emotional response of the analyst in the psychoanalytic situation. *International Journal of Psycho-Analysis 33*: 1-10.

Glover, J. (1926) Divergent tendencies in psychotherapy. *British Journal of Medical Psychology* 6: 93-109.

Glover, E. (1927). Lectures on Technique in Psycho-Analysis, IV – Countertransference and resistance. *International Journal of Psycho-Analysis* 8: 486-520.

Glover, E. (1928) The psychology of the psychotherapist *British Journal of Medical Psychology*. 9: 1-16,

Glover, E. (1935) *The Birth of the Ego: A Nuclear Hypothesis*. London: Allen and Unwin.

Glover, E. (1945) Examination of the Klein system of child psychology. P*sychoanalytic Study of the Child* 1: 75-118.

Gordon, J. and Kirtchuk, G. (Eds.) (2008) *Psychic Assaults and Frightened Clinicians*. London: Karnac.

Gottlieb, R.M. (1989) Technique and countertransference in Freud's analysis of the Rat Man. *Psychoanalysis Quarterly* 58: 29-62.

Green, A. (1983). The dead mother. In *On Private Madness*. Madison, CT: Int. Univ. Press, 1986, pp. 142-173.

Greenberg, J.R. (1991) Countertransference and reality. *Psychoanalytic Dialogues* 1: 52-73.

Greenberg, .J.R. and Mitchell, S. (1983) *Object Relations in Psychoanalytic Theory*. Cambridge, Mass: Harvard University Press.

Grosskurth, P. (1986) *Melanie Klein: Her World and her Work*. London: Hodder and Stoughton.

Hacking, I. 2001 *An Introduction to Probability and Inductive Logic*. Cambridge: Cambridge University Press.

Hanly, C. and Hanly, M.A. (2001) Critical Realism. *Journal of the American Psychoanalytic Association* 49:515-532.

Hardcastle, M, Kennard, D., Grandison, S., and Fagin, L. (Eds.) (2007) *Experiences of Mental Health In-Patient Care*. London: Routledge.

Hargreaves, E. and Varchevker, A. (Eds.) (2004) *In Pursuit of Psychic Change*. London: Routledge.

Hartmann, H. (1939) *Ego Psychology and the Problem of Adaptation*. New York: International Universities Press.

Haynal, A. (1999) The countertransference in the work of

Ferenczi. *American Journal of Psychoanalysis* 59: 315-331.

Heimann, P. (1943) Some Aspects of the Role of Introjection and Projection in Early Development. In King, P. and Steiner, R. (Eds.) (1991). The Freud–Klein Controversies 1941–45: 501-530. London: Routledge.

Heimann, P. (1950) On counter-transference. *International Journal of Psycho-Analysis 31*: 81-84. Republished in Paula Heimann (1989) *About Children and Children-No-Longer*, pp. 73-79. London: Routledge.

Heimann, P. (1952) Certain functions of projection and introjection in early infancy. In Klein. M., Heimann, P., Isaacs, S. and Riviere, J (Eds.) *Developments in Psychoanalysis*. London: Hogarth.

Heimann, P. (1960) Counter-transference. *British Journal of Medical Psychology 33:* 9-15. Republished in Paula Heimann (1989) *About Children and Children-No-Longer*: 151-160. London: Routledge.

Hinshelwood, R.D (1985) The patient's defensive analyst. *British Journal of Psychotherapy 2*: 30-41.

Hinshelwood, R. D. (1989) Little Hans' transference. *Journal of Child Psychotherapy 15*: 63-78.

Hinshelwood, R.D. (1997a) Transference and countertransference. In Burgoyne, Bernard and Sullivan, Mary (Eds.) *The Klein-Lacan Dialogues.* London: Rebus.

Hinshelwood, R.D. (1997b) The elusive concept of 'internal objects' and the origins of the Klein group 1934-1943. *International Journal of Psycho-Analysis 78*: 877-897.

Hinshelwood, R.D. (1997c) *Therapy or Coercion: Does Psycho-*Analysis *Differ from Brain-Washing?* London: Karnac.

Hinshelwood, R.D. (1999a) Countertransference. *International Journal of Psychoanalysis 80*: 797-818. Republished (2002) in Michels. R., Abensoour, L., Eizirik, C.L. and Rusbridger. R. (Eds.) *Key Papers on Countertransference.* London: Karnac.

Hinshelwood, R.D. (1999b) The difficult patient: the role of 'scientific' psychiatry in understanding patients with chronic schizophrenia or severe personality disorder. *British Journal of Psychiatry 14*: 187-190.

Hinshelwood, R.D. and Skogstad, W. (eds.) 2000 *Observing Organisations.* London: Routledge.

Hinshelwood, R.D. (2001a) Concluding reflections: surveying the maze. In Serge Frisch, R.D. Hinshelwood and Jean-Marie Gauthier (eds) *Psychoanalysis and Psychotherapy: The Controversies and the Future.* London: Karnac.

Hinshelwood, R.D. (2001b) *Thinking about Institutions. Milieux and Madness.* London: Jessica Kingsley.

Hinshelwood, R.D. (2004) *Suffering Insanity: Three Psychoanalytic Essays on Psychosis.* London: Routledge.

Hinshelwood, R.D. (2007) The Kleinian theory of therapeutic action. *Psychoanalytic Quarterly 76* (supplement): 1479-1498.

Hinshelwood, R.D. (2008) Melanie Klein and countertransference: a historical note. *Psychoanalysis and History 10*: 95-113.

Hinshelwood, R.D. (2009) Do unconscious processes affect educational institutions? *Clinical Child Psychology and Psychiatry 14*: 509-522.

Hinshelwood, R.D. (2010) Psychoanalytic research: Is clinical material any use? *Psychoanalytic Psychotherapy 24*: 362–379.

Hinshelwood, R.D. (2013a) *Research on the Couch: Subjectivity, Single Case Studies and Psychoanalytic Knowledge.* London: Routledge.

Hinshelwood, R.D. (2013b) Freud's countertransference. In Oelsner, R. (Ed.) *Transference and Countertransference.* London: Routledge.

Hinshelwood, R.D. 2014 Projection and Introjection: The uses of paternalism, and its abuses. OUP *Online Handbook of Psychiatric Ethics*. Oxford: OUP.

Hoffman, I.Z. and Gill, M.M. (1988) Critical reflections on a coding scheme. *International Journal of Psycho-Analysis 69*: 55-64.

Isaacs, S. (1939) Criteria for interpretation. *International Journal of Psycho-Analysis 20*: 148-160.

Isaacs, S. (1948) The nature and function of phantasy. *International Journal of Psycho-Analysis* 29:73-97. Original version (1943) in King, P. and Steiner, R. (1991). The Freud–Klein Controversies 1941–45: 264-321. London: Routledge.

Jaques, Elliot (1955) Social systems as a defence against persecutory and depressive anxiety. In: Klein, Heimann & Money-Kyrle (Eds.) *New Directions in Psycho-Analysis*; 478-498. London: Tavistock

Jelliffe, S.E. (1930). British Journal of Medical Psychology. *Psychoanalytic Review 17*: 348-359,

Jones, Ernest (1935) Early female sexuality. *International Journal of Psychoanalysis 16*:263-273.

Joseph, B. (1975) The patient who is difficult to reach. In P L Giovacchini (Ed.) *Tactics and Techiques in Psycho-Analytic Therapy, Volume 2, Counter-Transference*. New York: Jason Aronson. Republished in Betty Joseph (1989) *Psychic Equilibrium and Psychic Change*. London: Routledge.

Joseph, B. (1978) Different types of anxiety and their handling in the analytic situation. *International Journal of Psychoanalysis 59*: 223-228.

Joseph, B. (1987) Projective identification: some clinical aspects. In Sandler J. (Ed.) *Projection, Identification, Projective Identification*. Madison, CT: International Universities Press: 65-76. Republished (1989) in *Psychic Equilibrium and Psychic Change*: 168-180. London and New York: Routledge.

Joseph, B. (1988). Object relations in clinical practice, *Psychoanalytic. Quarterly 57*: 626-642. Republished in *Psychic Equilibrium and Psychic Change*: 203-215. London: Routledge

Joseph, B. (1989) *Psychic Equilibrium and Psychic Change*. London: Routledge.

Kierkegaard, S. (1989 [1841]) *Kierkegaard's Writings, II: The Concept of Irony, with Continual Reference to Socrates*. New Jersey: Princeton University Press.

King, P. (1978) Affective Responses of the Analyst to the Patient's Communications. *International Journal of Psycho-Analysis 76*: 723-738.

King, P. and Steiner, R. (1991). The Freud–Klein Controversies 1941–45. London: Routledge.

Kirsner, D. (1999) *Unfree Associations: Inside Psychoanalytic Institutions*. London: Process Press.

Klein, M. (1943) Memorandum on her technique. In King, P. and Steiner, R. (eds) (1991) *The Freud-Klein Controversies, 1941-1945*: 635-638. London: Routledge.

Klein, M. (1946) Notes on some schizoid mechanisms', *International Journal of Psycho-Analysis 27*: 99-110. Republished (1975) in *The Writings of Melanie Klein, Volume 3*: 1-24. London: Hogarth.

Klein, M. (1952 [1946]) Notes on some schizoid mechanisms, In Melanie Klein, Paula Heimann, Susan Isaacs and Joan Riviere, *Developments in Psycho-Analysis*. London: Hogarth: 292-320. Republished in T*he Writings of Melanie Klein, Volume 3*: 247-263. *London Hogarth*.

Klein, M. (1959) Our adult world and its roots in infancy. *Human Relations 12*: 291-303. Republished 1963 in *Our Adult World and Other Essays*. London: Heinemann. Republished in T*he Writings of Melanie Klein, Volume 3*:

247-263. *London Hogarth.*

Kohon,G. (1986) *The British School of Psychoanalysis.* London: Free Association Books.

Kohut, H. (1971) *The Analysis of the Self: A Systematic Approach to the Psychoanalytic Treatment of Narcissistic Personality Disorders* New York: International Universities Press.

Laing, R.D. (1960) *The Divided Self: A Study in Sanity and Madness.* London: Tavistock.

Lamb, S. D. (2014) *Pathologist of the Mind: Adolf Meyer and the Origins of American Psychiatry.* Baltimore: Johns Hopkins University Press.

Levenson, E.A. (1984) Harry Stack Sullivan – *The web and the spider. Contemporary Psychoanalysis 20*: 174-188.

Leuzinger-Bohleber, M. and Target, M. (Eds.) (2002) *Outcomes of Psychoanalytic Treatment.* London: Whurr.

LeBon, G. (1895) *Psychologie des foules.* Paris: Alcan. English translation, (1995) as *The Crowd.* London: Transaction Publishers.

Litowitz, B.E. (2002). Continuity and change in psychoanalytic theory. *Journal of the American Psychoanalysis Association 50*: 13-17.

Little, M. (1951) Counter-transference and the patient's response to it. *International Journal of Psycho-Analysis 32*: 32-40.

Mahony, P. (1986) *Freud and the Ratman.* New Haven: Yale University Press.

Main, T. (1975) Some psychodynamics of large groups. In Kreeger, L. (ed) The Large Group: 57-86. London: Constable. Republished (1989) in Main, T.F. *The Ailment and other Psychoanalytic Essays.* London: Free Association Books.

McGuire, W. (1974) *The Freud/Jung Letters.* London: Hogarth.

Meares, R. (1993). *The Metaphor of Play.* Northvale, NJ: Jason Aronson

Menzies Lyth, I. (1959) The functioning of social systems as a defence against anxiety: a report on a study of the nursing service of a general hospital. *Human Relations 13*: 95-121. Republished (1988) in Menzies *Containing Anxiety in Institutions.* London: Free Association Books; and in Trist and Murray (Eds.) (1990) *The Social Engagement of Social Science.* London: Free Association Books.

Menzies Lyth, I. (1988) *Containing Anxiety in Institutions.* London: Free Association Books.

Milgram, S. (1964) Group pressure and action against a person. *Journal of Abnormal and Social Psychology 64*: 137-43.

Miller, E. and Gwynne, G. (1972) *A Life Apart*. London: Tavistock.

Milner, M. (1952) Aspects of symbolism in comprehension of the not-self. *International Journal of Psychoanalysis 33*: 181-194.

Mitchell, S. A. (1988) *Relational Concepts in Psychoanalysis*. Cambridge, MA: Harvard University Press.

Mitchell, S. (1993). *Hope and Dread in Psychoanalysis*. New York: Basic Books.

Money-Kyrle, R. (1956) Normal counter-transference and some of its deviations. *International Journal of Psychoanalysis 37*: 360-366. Republished (1978) in *The Collected Papers of Roger Money-Kyrle*. Perthshire: Clunie Press. And republished in Elizabeth Spillius (1988) *Melanie Klein Today, Volume 2 – Mainly Practice*. London: Routledge.

Nagel, T. (1974) What is it like to be a bat? *Philosophical Review*. 83: 435-50.

Nash, O. (1935) Professional men. In *I Wouldn't Have Missed It: Selected Poems of Ogden Nash* (1975). New York: Little, Brown.

Norton, K. and Hinshelwood, R.D. (1996) Severe personality disorder: treatment issues and selection for in-patient psychotherapy. *British Journal of Psychiatry 168*: 723-731.

Ochberg, F. 1978 The victim of terrorism: Psychiatric considerations. *Journal of Conflict and Terrorism 1*: 147-168.

Ogden, T.H. (1988). On the dialectical structure of experience – *Some Clinical and Theoretical Implications. Contemporary Psychoanalysis 24*: 17-45.

Ogden, T.H. (1994) *Subjects of Analysis.* London: Karnac.

Ogden, T.H. (1995). Analysing forms of aliveness and deadness of the transference-countertransference. *International Journal of Psychoanalysis 76*: 695-709.

Ogden, T.H. (1996). Reconsidering three aspects of psychoanalytic technique. *International Journal of Psychoanalysis 77*: 883-899.

Ogden, T. (1999) The analytic third: an overview. In Mitchell, S and Aron, L. (Eds.), *Relational Perspectives in Psychoanalysis: The Emergence of a Tradition*: 487-492). Hillsdale, NJ: Analytic Press.

Ogden, T.H. (2004). The analytic third. *Psychoanalytic Quarterly 73*: 167-195.

Orange, D. (1995 *Emotional Understanding*. New York: Guilford.

O'shaughnessy, E. (1992) Enclaves and excursions. *International Journal of Psycho-Analysis*, *73*: 603-611

O'Shaughnessy, E. (1983) Words and working through. *International Journal of Psycho-Analysis 64*: 281-289.

Peräkylä, A. (2010) Shifting the perspective after the patient's response to an interpretation. *International Journal of Psycho-Analysis 91*:1363-1384.

Pines. Malcolm (1978) Group analytic psychotherapy with borderline personality disorder. *Group Analysis 11*: 115-126.

Poland, Warren (2000) The analyst's witnessing and otherness. *Journal of the American Psychoanalytic Association 48*: 17-34.

Quinodoz, J.-M. (2009) *Listening to Hanna Segal: Her Contribution to Psychoanalysis*. London: Routledge.

Racker, H. (1953). A Contribution to the Problem of Counter-Transference. *International Journal of Psychoanalysis 34*: 313-324.

Racker, H. (1968) *Transference and Countertransference*. London: Hogarth.

Raynor, Eric (1991) *The Independent Mind in British Psychoanalysis*. London: Free Association Books.

Reich, A. (1951) On counter-transference. *International Journal of Psycho-Analysis 32*: 25-31.

Renik, O. (1993a) Countertransference enactment and the psychoanalytic process. In: *Psychic Structure and Psychic Change. Essays in Honor of Robert S. Wallerstein*: 135-158. Madison, CT: International Universities Press.

Renik, O. (1993b) Analytic interaction: conceptualizing technique in light of the analyst's irreducible subjectivity. *Psychoanalysis Quarterly 62*: 553-571.

Renik, Owen (1998) The Analyst's Subjectivity and the Analyst's Objectivity. *International Journal of Psycho-Analysis 79*: 487-497.

Renik, Owen (1999) Renik replies to Cavell. *International Journal of Psycho-Analysis 80*: 382-383.

Richards, A. D. and Richards, A. K. (1995) Notes on psychoanalytic theory and its consequences for technique. *Journal of Clinical Psychoanalysis 4*: 429-456.

Riviere, J. (1936) On the genesis of psychical conflict in earliest infancy. *International Journal of Psychoanalysis 17*:395-422

Rosenfeld, H. (1987) *Impasse and Interpretation*. London: Routledge.

Rudnytsky, P.L. (1999) 'Does the Professor Talk to God?': Countertransference and Jewish identity in the case of Little Hans. *Psychoanalysis and History 1*: 175-194.

Sandler, J. (1976) Countertransference and role-responsiveness. *International Review of Psychoanalysis* 3:43-47.

Sandler, J. (1983) Reflections on some relations between psychoanalytic concepts and psychoanalytic practice. *International Journal of Psycho-Analysis 64*: 35-44.

Sandler, J. (1993) On communication from patient to analyst: Not everything is projective identification. *International Journal of Psychoanalysis 74*: 1097-1107.

Sandler, J. and Sandler, A. (1987) The past unconscious, the present unconscious and the vicissitudes of guilt. *International Journal of Psychoanalysis 68*: 331-341.

Schafer, R. (1997). Vicissitudes of remembering in the countertransference. *International Journal of Psychoanalysis 78*: 1151-1163.

Schwaber, E.A. (1996) The conceptualisation and communication of clinical facts in psychoanalysis: A discussion. *International Journal of Psychoanalysis 77*: 235-253.

Searles, H. (1979) *Countertransference and Related Subjects: Selected Papers*. New York: International Universities Press.

Segal, H. (1975) A psycho-analytic approach to the treatment of psychoses. In M.H. Lader (Ed.), *Studies in Schizophrenia*, Ashford: Headley. Reprinted (1981 in *The Work of Hanna Segal*, New York: Jason Aronson.

Segal, H. 1981 The function of dreams. In *Do I Dare Disturb the Universe*: 579-587 (Ed.) Grotstein, J. Beverly Hills: Caesura Press.

Segal, H. (1991). *Dream, Phantasy, and Art*. London/New York: Tavistock-Routledge.

Spillius, E. (1988) *Melanie Klein Today, Volumes 1 and 2*. London: Routledge.

Spillius, E. (1992) Clinical experiences of projective identification. In Robin Anderson (Ed.) *Clinical Lectures on Klein and Bion*. London: Routledge.

Spillius, E. (2007) *Encounters with Melanie Klein*. London: Routledge.

Steiner, J. (1993) Problems of psychoanalytic technique: Patient-centred and analyst-centred interpretations. In *Psychic Retreats*: 131-146. London: Routledge.

Stewart, H. (1996). *Michael Balint object relations pure and applied.* London: Routledge.

Stewart, H. (1977). Problems of management in the analysis of a hallucinating hysteric. *International Journal of Psycho-Analysis* 38: 67-76

Strachey, J. (1934) The nature of the therapeutic action of psychoanalysis. *International Journal of Psycho-Analysis* 15: 127-159. Republished (1969) *International Journal of Psycho-Analysis* 50: 275-192.

Sullivan, H.S. (1953) *The Interpersonal Theory of Psychiatry.* New York: Norton.¹

Symington, N. (1983). The analyst's act of freedom as agent of therapeutic change. *International Journal of Psycho-Analysis* 10: 283-291

Tonnesmann, M. (1989) Editor's introduction. In Heimann, P. *About Children and Children-no-Longer: Collected Papers 1942-1980.* London: Routledge.

Tuckett, D. (1994) The conceptualisation and communication of clinical facts in psychoanalysis – Foreword. *International Journal of Psycho-Analysis* 75: 865-870.

Tuckett, D., Basile, R., Birkstead-Breen, D., Bohm, T. Denis, P., Ferro, A., Hinz, H., Jemstedt, A., Mariotti, P.anad

Schubert, J. (2008) *Psychoanalysis Comparable and Incomparable: The Evolution of a Method.* London: Routledge.

Waelder, R. (1937). The problem of the genesis of psychical conflict in earliest infancy. *International Journal of Psychoanalysis* 18:406-473.

Wheelis, A. (1956) The vocational hazards of psycho-analysis. *International Journal of Psychoanalysis* 37:171-184.

Winnicott, D.W. (1945) Primitive emotional development. *International Journal of Psychoanalysis* 26: 137-143.

Winnicott, D.W. (1949) Hate in the countertransference. *International Journal of Psychoanalysis* 30: 69-74. Republished (1958) in *Through Paediatrics to Psychoanalysis.* London: Tavistock.

Winnicott, D.W. (1955) Metapsychological and clinical aspects of regression within the psycho-analytical set-up. *International Journal of Psychoanalysis* 36: 16-26.

Winnicott, D.W. (1960) The theory of the parent-infant relationship. *International Journal of Psychoanalysis* 41:585-595.

Winnicott, D.W. (1969) The use of an object. *International Journal of Psycho-Analysis* 50: 711-716.

Winnicott, D.W. (1971) *Playing and Reality. London: Tavistock.*

Zetzel, E.R. (1956). Current concepts of transference. *International Journal of Psychoanalysis* 37: 369-375.

9 781899 209170